The Handbook of Biological Therapy

The Handbook of Biological Therapy

A guide to the use and safety of biological therapies in Rheumatology, Dermatology, and Gastroenterology

Bruce Kirkham
Professor of Rheumatology
University of New South Wales, Sydney

Arthur Kavanaugh
Professor of Medicine
University of California, San Diego
Department of Rheumatology, Allergy and Immunology

Jonathan Barker
Professor and Director
St John's Institute of Dermatology
St Thomas' Hospital, London

Scott Plevy
Associate Professor of Medicine,
Microbiology and Immunology
University of North Carolina School of Medicine

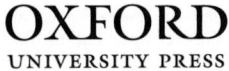

OXFORD
UNIVERSITY PRESS

Great Clarendon Street, Oxford OX2 6DP

Oxford University Press is a department of the University of Oxford.
It furthers the University's objective of excellence in research, scholarship,
and education by publishing worldwide in

Oxford New York

Auckland Cape Town Dar es Salaam Hong Kong Karachi
Kuala Lumpur Madrid Melbourne Mexico City Nairobi
New Delhi Shanghai Taipei Toronto

With offices in

Argentina Austria Brazil Chile Czech Republic France Greece
Guatemala Hungary Italy Japan Poland Portugal Singapore
South Korea Switzerland Thailand Turkey Ukraine Vietnam

Oxford is a registered trade mark of Oxford University Press
in the UK and in certain other countries

Published in the United States
by Oxford University Press Inc., New York

© Oxford University Press 2008

The moral rights of the author have been asserted
Database right Oxford University Press (maker)

First published 2008

All rights reserved. No part of this publication may be reproduced,
stored in a retrieval system, or transmitted, in any form or by any means,
without the prior permission in writing of Oxford University Press,
or as expressly permitted by law, or under terms agreed with the appropriate
reprographics rights organization. Enquiries concerning reproduction
outside the scope of the above should be sent to the Rights Department,
Oxford University Press, at the address above

You must not circulate this book in any other binding or cover
and you must impose this same condition on any acquirer

British Library Cataloguing in Publication Data

Data available

Library of Congress Cataloguing in Publication Data

Data available

Typeset by Cepha Imaging Private Ltd., Bangalore, India
Printed and bound in the
United Kingdom
by Ashford Colour Press Ltd, Gosport, Hampshire

ISBN 978–0–19–920816–6

10 9 8 7 6 5 4 3 2

Whilst every effort has been made to ensure that the contents of this book are as
complete, accurate and up-to-date as possible at the date of writing, Oxford
University Press is not able to give any guarantee or assurance that such is the case.
Readers are urged to take appropriately qualified medical advice in all cases. The
information in this book is intended to be useful to the general reader, but should
not be used as a means of self-diagnosis or for the prescription of medication.

Foreword

I wholeheartedly recommend this handbook to clinicians who prescribe products of the biotechnology industry to treat chronic inflammatory diseases. Biologic agents have created milestones in the history of rheumatology, dermatology, and gastroenterology. Various aspects of diseases that caused a major burden for the affected patients could be treated in a way unseen before. In addition many patient-centred aspects of the disease improved such as fatigue and possibilities to continue a normal lifestyle. These new interventions appeared to be safer than all researchers who participated in the early days of their development expected. Nevertheless considerable insight on occurring side effects has been obtained and solid clinical research provided standards of optimal monitoring and preventive actions to avoid major side effects.

As with all new therapies in health care, the introduction of these agents was relatively slow. In the case of biologic agents the introduction was also complicated by the new way of administration and the costs involved. Now we have reached a point where no practice operates without the application of these agents. The practising physician is confronted with many questions from patients, colleagues, health professionals, and administrators. In addition, this class of drugs is associated with pharmacological principles that need to be understood given the fact that the introduction of many more biologic agents can be expected. Despite the breakthrough of the currently available drugs targeting cytokines and lymphocytes, there is still an unmet need that hopefully can be treated with agents that can be expected in the near future. For these reasons this book edited by Kirkham, Kavanaugh, Barker, and Plevy provides precisely the information needed by clinicians. The information contained in it provides a comprehensive overview of the knowledge essential for clinical practice and education.

Ferry Breedveld
Professor of Rheumatology
President of EULAR

Preface

Drugs produced by molecular biological techniques, called the 'biologics', differ from the usual chemical medications. Firstly, they are all proteins, either monoclonal antibodies or fusion proteins, with different pharmacokinetic and patient response characteristics. Secondly, their unique specificity of action produces unique adverse events related to their ability to neutralize specific immune pathways. Many adverse events are due to suppression of normal immune mechanisms of host defence or immune tolerance. They challenge the practising clinician with a range of judgements for optimal use and detection and management of adverse events. This new collection of screening strategies and adverse events is outside the normal range usually found with the small-molecule chemical therapeutics commonly used to date.

Tumour necrosis factor (TNF) blocking therapy (TNF-blockers) is an important new class of biologic therapy for rheumatoid arthritis, ankylosing spondylitis, Crohn's disease, ulcerative colitis, psoriasis, and psoriatic arthritis. The introduction of TNF-blockers was unusual in that the initial pre-licensing clinical trials involved small numbers of patients, and much of the experience of unusual toxicities and dose manipulation has been gained from postmarketing studies. This class of drugs is now being used increasingly around the world. This increased use will require knowledge of these drugs by primary care practitioners who are involved in the day-to-day care of these patients, in addition to the specialist prescribers.

Additional biological drugs such as abatacept and rituximab, and a new TNF-blocker, have recently received licences for some indications. These new drugs will have new idiosyncratic adverse events that necessitate more information for the clinician. Intensive research is also defining new areas in which these drugs will be used in the future, increasing the number of practitioners using biologics.

The aim of this book is to provide the practising clinician with a practical guide to the use of these drugs in the setting of daily practice. We believe it will provide a comprehensive distillation of the clinical experience with these drugs, combined with data from diverse databases to provide practical information about their use in daily practice. This book has been designed to be practical, and as such it does not cover the modes of action of the different biologics in detail. In addition to covering common adverse events, we hope to provide information about infrequent but important clinical questions that make the use of these drugs difficult for the busy practitioner. All of the authors have been involved with these drugs from the beginnings of the clinical trial programmes, and continue to use them in daily practice.

We hope the book will be useful for every clinician who treats patients with biologics and assist in answering the questions that arise every day.

Bruce Kirkham
Arthur Kavanaugh
Jonathan Barker
Scott Plevy

Contents

Foreword *v*
Preface *vii*

TNF – tumour necrosis factor α *xi*
Mode of action of anti-TNF *xii*
TNF-blocking drugs in clinical use *xiii*
TNF-blocking drugs not in clinical use *xiv*

Section 1 **TNF-blocker safety**

Increased risk of infection *2*
Tuberculosis *3*
Opportunistic infections *7*
Injection-site reactions *7*
Allergic, hypersensitivity reactions, anaphylactic responses *7*
Psoriasis *8*
Infusion reactions (infliximab) *8*
Malignancy and lymphoproliferative conditions *9*
Drug-induced lupus-like reactions *12*
Anti-drug antibodies (immunogenicity) *12*
Congestive heart failure *13*
Neurological *14*
Hepatobiliary *15*
Use in pregnancy *16*
Lactation *17*
Respiratory *17*
Vaccinations *17*
Use of TNF-blockers with other medications *18*
Haematological *18*
Postmarketing safety experience in Crohn's disease *18*

Section 2 Rheumatology

Rheumatoid arthritis 27

Other rheumatological conditions 34

TNF-blocking therapy in ankylosing spondylitis and psoriatic arthritis 38

Ankylosing spondylitis 38

Psoriatic arthritis 44

Adalimumab (Humira) 48

Etanercept (Enbrel) 57

Infliximab (Remicade) 68

Certolizumab pegol (Cimzia) 79

Abatacept (Orencia) 81

Anakinra (Kineret) 89

B-cell depletion: Rituximab (Rituxan® [USA], MabThera® [Europe, Asia, South America]) 93

Section 3 Dermatology

Psoriasis 98

Approaches to management 99

Assessing disease severity 100

Important differences between psoriasis and rheumatoid arthritis 101

Biological therapy for psoriasis 101

Etanercept (Enbrel) 103

Infliximab (Remicade) 106

Adalimumab (Humira) 110

Efalizumab (Raptiva) 113

Alefacept (Amevive) 118

Section 4 Gastroenterology

Biological therapy in inflammatory bowel disease and Crohn's disease 122

Adalimumab (Humira) 131

Infliximab (Remicade) 135

Natalizumab (Tysabri) 143

Certolizumab pegol (Cimzia) 148

Index 151

TNF – tumour necrosis factor α

Tumour necrosis factor (TNF) is made up of three identical subunits forming a homotrimer. It functions in two forms, soluble and cell surface expressed.

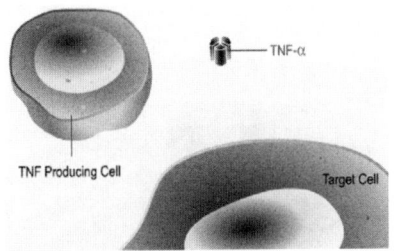

Soluble TNF

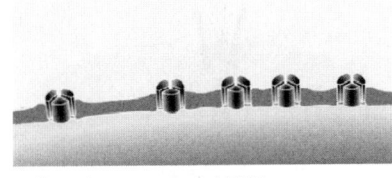

Cell-surface-expressed TNF

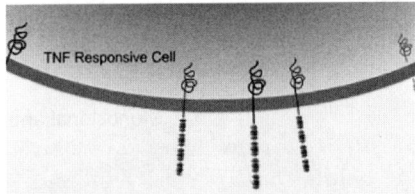

TNF activates cells by binding and cross-linking TNF receptors on the cell surface. There are two receptors, TNFR1 (p55) and TNFR2 (p75)

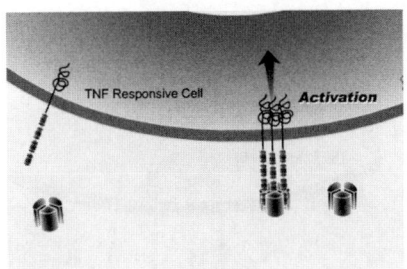

Activation by soluble TNF

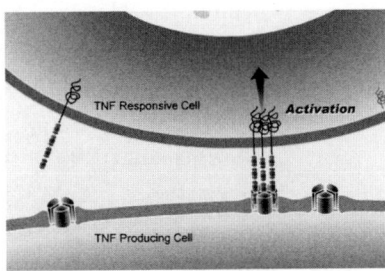

Activation by cell surface TNF

The activation of one or the other of these different receptors by different mechanisms produces various immunological responses.

Mode of action of anti-TNF

Soluble TNF is bound and neutralized by both receptor constructs and monoclonal antibodies.

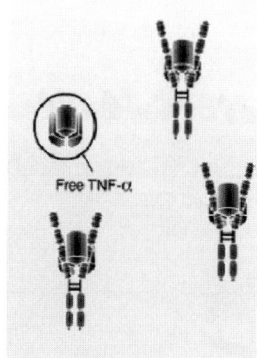

Receptor constructs

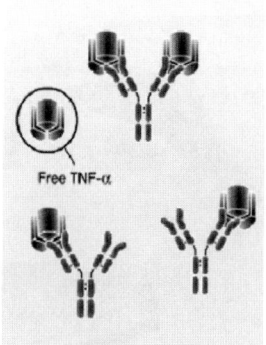

Monoclonal antibodies

Receptor constructs can also bind and neutralize TNFβ (otherwise known as lymphotoxin α).

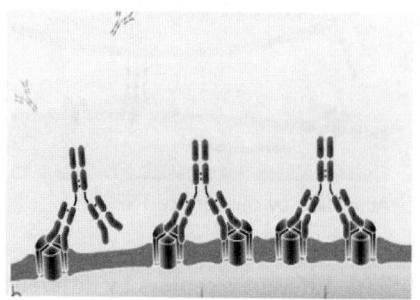
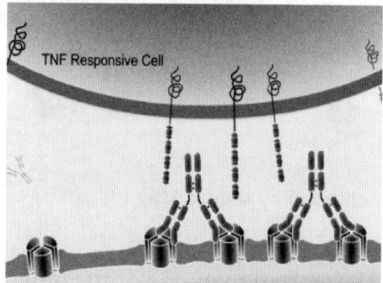

Cell-surface-expressed TNF is bound and neutralized better by monoclonal antibodies.

TNF-blocking drugs in clinical use

Adalimumab

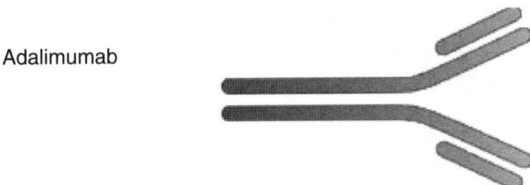

Human anti-TNF monoclonal antibody made by phage display techniques

Infliximab

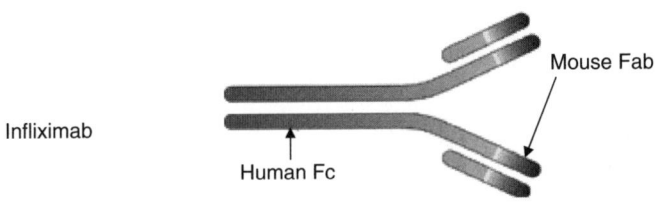

Chimaeric human–mouse monoclonal antibody

Etanercept

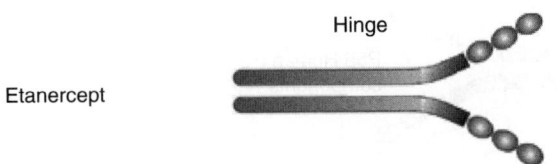

P75 receptor construct attached to human Fc via a hinge region

Certolizumab pegol

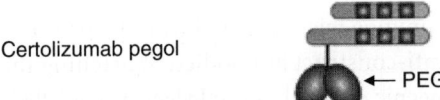

Polyethylene glycol (PEG) attached to a humanized Fab fragment

TNF-blocking drugs not in clinical use

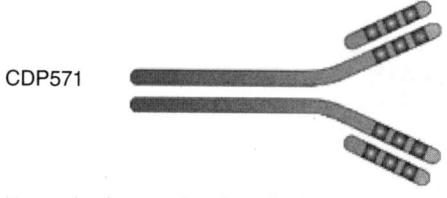

CDP571

Humanized monoclonal antibody

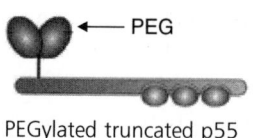

PEGylated truncated p55

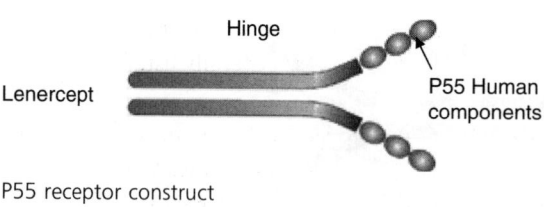

Lenercept

P55 receptor construct

P55 receptor constructs are very immunogenic compared with the p75 constructs, producing high levels of anti-construct antibodies. Shortening the construct and covering the immunogenic end with polyethylene glycol (PEG) reduces this response.

1
TNF-blocker safety

Biological therapy with TNF inhibitors has radically changed the treatment of refractory inflammatory arthritis, bowel disease, and psoriasis. The use of TNF-blockers has become an integral part in the management of these conditions [1–4]. Short- and long-term therapy with TNF inhibitors is well tolerated; however, the increased risk of infrequent but serious complications, such as opportunistic infection, autoimmunity, infusion reactions, and lymphoma, warrant sustained vigilance on the part of physicians and patients alike. The decision to initiate and continue therapy must be based on weighing the risk of complications versus benefit to the patient and is paramount in the ability of the physician to utilize biological therapies to their fullest potential [5,6].

Safety data for TNF-blockers was initially obtained from the clinical trials programme in many different indications. These early data have been supplemented extensively by information from postmarketing databases, some of which have compared patients on TNF-blocker therapy with patients receiving non-biological immunosuppressive therapies [7–10]. The current consensus is that most safety issues are relevant to the class of TNF-blockers, i.e. the antibodies and the receptor construct. For this reason, safety will be presented for the TNF-blockers as a class, with comments to identify any drug-specific issues. Most data have been derived from patients with rheumatoid arthritis (RA) and Crohn's disease. The adverse events are generally listed in order of severity and frequency.

In RA, preliminary data from long-term large databases show that patients receiving TNF-blocker therapy have lower mortality rates than those not receiving them [8]. These types of study, however, are prone to artefacts, particularly that of confounding by indication. In this situation, patients do or do not have a specific therapy because of disease or co-morbidity factors that influence the long-term outcome independently of any effect of the intervention under study. In the case of TNF-blockers it may be expected that patients with poor respiratory reserve, frequent infections, and diabetes or cardiac failure would not receive these drugs. Therefore, the comparison groups must have assessments of pre-existing co-morbidity before clear judgements of safety can be made.

Increased risk of infection

TNF plays an important role in cellular immunity, especially granuloma formation in infectious diseases caused by intracellular microorganisms such as *Mycobacterium tuberculosis*, *Listeria*, *Histoplasma*, or *Coccidioides* [11]. Large controlled trials of infliximab for patients with Crohn's disease have reported serious infections in up to 4.6% of patients. Open-label trials and retrospective studies have revealed increased opportunistic infections, such as tuberculosis, listeriosis, and histoplasmosis [12]. Likewise, in patients with RA, TNF blockade increases the risk of the above infections in patients taking disease-modifying antirheumatic drugs (DMARDs), such as methotrexate, sulfasalazine and leflunomide. In RA, long-term databases indicate that the most frequently increased incidence is of cellulitis, upper respiratory tract infection (URTI) and pneumonia [7–10]. Bacterial infections can occur at all known sites (e.g. pneumonia, pyelonephritis, septic arthritis). These occur on a background of increased infections in patients with RA compared with normal subjects. Data from the British Society for Rheumatology Biologics Registry (BSRBR) also show little difference in the incidence of common infections between the three currently used TNF-blockers [10]. Further analysis of this database suggests that infections are increased, particularly within the first 3 months of therapy [13].

The Dutch experience comparing serious infection (leading to either hospitalization or death) rates in patients after starting their third DMARD versus TNF-blockers shows an increased rate of serious infections, especially pneumonia, skin or joint infections: 2.76 versus 1.65 per 100 patient-years, rate ratio 1.68 (95% confidence interval (CI) 1.23–2.30) [14].

The START (**S**afety **T**rial for Rheumatoid **A**rthritis with **R**emicade [Infliximab] **T**herapy) study of dose-related safety of infliximab therapy for RA demonstrated that infection rates of infliximab at doses of 3 and 5 mg/kg were not significantly different from those in placebo-treated patients, although the incidence of infections was significantly increased in patients receiving 10 mg/kg [7].

In the Research in Active Rheumatoid Arthritis (ReAct) trial of adalimumab in RA [15], with 6610 patients (median follow-up time 211 days, maximum 669 days) representing 4210 patient-years of adalimumab exposure, serious infections were reported in 202 patients. Independent predictors were preexisting pulmonary and cardiac disease, male sex, higher screening disability (HAQ-DI) score and increased age.

The question of any increased risk of infection in the perioperative period in patients receiving TNF-blocker therapy is unclear. Recent reports show either no increased risk [16,17], or significant increased risk [18].

Tuberculosis

Tuberculosis (TB) infections are significantly increased in patients receiving TNF-blockers compared with other groups receiving immunosuppressive therapy [19,20]. Tuberculosis infections are more common in patients receiving antibodies than in those receiving the receptor construct [21]. This may be due in part to different populations exposed to the TNF-blockers, but may also be a consequence of differences in the properties of the antibodies compared with the receptor construct. However, TB occurs with all TNF-blockers [22–24], and the advice is to screen and monitor all patients in a similar way.

TNF plays a critical role in the continuous process of suppressing latent TB. Most cases of TB are due to reactivation of latent TB, which has been present for years in a clinically dormant state. Compared with non-biologic-treated populations there is an increased rate of non-pulmonary TB (lymph node, abdominal). There have also been cases of patients on TNF-blocking therapy developing TB, probably as a result of recent exposure to new TB infection.

The surveillance for TB has several steps.

Screening for latent TB

Policies for screening have been made in many countries and these should be followed. Current recommendations by the British Thoracic Society warrant a thorough history, clinical examination, a tuberculin skin test if appropriate and, if indicated, chest radiography (CXR) to evaluate for tuberculosis exposure before initiating anti-TNF therapy [25]. The history is very important and needs to ascertain whether the patient was exposed to TB as a child, has lived in an endemic area, or has other risks for exposure to TB such as alcoholism or drug addiction, human immunodeficincy virus (HIV) infection, and exposure to TB in workplaces such as hospitals, or social exposure such as jails or homeless shelters [26].

The following tests are used:

Tuberculin purified protein derivative (PPD) skin testing The skin test must be performed by personnel experienced in the application and assessment of the skin changes after 48 hours, with the skin induration (thickening) diameter of 5 mm indicating latent TB. Other disadvantages relate to reduced skin recall antigen reactivity in active inflammatory diseases and in patients receiving immunosuppressive therapy, making the test less sensitive. The reduction of skin reaction diameter from 10 to 5 mm is made to correct for this. The influence of previous BCG vaccination on the result is controversial, especially in adults immunized in childhood. The test is relatively cheap, although reagents can be difficult to access at times. In Europe, the Heaf skin test is sometimes preferred and should used in a similar way.

Chest radiography (X-ray) This is used for signs of previous or currently active pulmonary TB. The test is cheap, readily available, and provides background information on CXR status for future comparison. It is thought by many experts to be very insensitive, and will not detect non-pulmonary latent TB.

Blood tests for TB reactivity Two different tests measure peripheral blood lymphocyte reactivity to *Mycobacterium tuberculosis* and therefore are not confounded by previous BCG vaccination. The tests require access to laboratory facilities, and the resolution of their place in screening patients receiving TNF-blockers is still in process. However, large experience in HIV medicine suggests that both tests are sensitive and specific. The tests are undergoing improvements and the place of these new-generation tests is being assessed in development studies of TNF-blockers, many in regions with higher background rates of TB compared with Europe and North America.

These procedures all have logistical, expense and sensitivity issues. The relevance of which tests are most appropriate depends on background population characteristics such as rates of TB and use of BCG vaccination, which, together with local resource availability, make the use of local guidelines very important.

The usefulness of a screening process is illustrated by the experience in Spain in the treatment of RA. A rate of active TB 22.6-fold higher than the Spanish population background rates and 6.2-fold higher than a comparator RA population not receiving TNF-blockers (EMECAR [Morbidity and Clinical Expression of Rheumatoid Arthritis] (Study) group) was experienced early in the use of TNF-blockers. Screening procedures for latent TB were mandatory PPD skin testing, which included a repeat skin test for patients with an initial negative response of less than 5 mm and CXR for all patients prior to initiation of TNF-blocking therapy. After initiation of this comprehensive screening strategy, the rate of TB fell by 83% and reached the EMECAR rate (IRR [incidence risk ratio] 1.0, 95% CI 0.02–8.2) [27].

Response to identification of latent TB

If the patient is identified to have currently active TB, this should be treated appropriately by an experienced physician with multiple anti-TB drug therapy, depending on local best practice. Currently, most authorities recommend that TNF-blocking therapy should not be instituted until the patient has successfully completed a full course of anti-TB therapy.

If tests indicate latent TB, or in high-risk patients, and if TNF-blocking therapy is still indicated after a discussion of risk/benefit with the patient, limited anti-TB prophylactic treatment with isoniazid (INH) or combination rifampicin–isoniazid therapy, depending on local TB sensitivities, is recommended. The length of treatment depends on local guidelines, but should be at least 6 months for isoniazid monotherapy, and 3 months has been suggested for combination isoniazid–rifampicin.

TNF-blocking therapy can usually be initiated after the patient has received treatment for latent TB for at least 1 month, although this recommendation has never been tested rigorously [28,29]. Patients receiving latent TB prophylaxis need to be monitored for adverse events, especially for abnormal liver function. Initial reports suggesting an increased risk of abnormal liver function in patients receiving methotrexate have not been supported by more recent US studies [30,31]. The combination of isoniazid–rifampicin is associated with a slightly higher rate of abnormal liver function test (LFT) results. It is important to establish a close liaison with a specialist in TB when dealing with patients with latent infections or reactivation during the course of anti-TNF therapy [32].

Registries from countries with long experience of TNF-blocker use report a continued low incidence of TB in patients receiving TNF-blocker therapy many years after beginning treatment [24].

An update of the Spanish experience of the impact of the new strict screening guidelines introduced in 2002 from the BIOBADASER – Spanish Society of Rheumatology Database on Biologic Products – database was reported in 2007 [33]. Some 5198 patients were registered, with 15 cases of TB (8 IFX – infliximab, 4 ADAL – adalimumab, 3 ETN – etanercept), nine within 5 months of treatment. Only one patient with TB had the complete screening protocol, with only five patients having repeat skin tests after an initial negative test, with four tests negative and the remaining one positive case not being treated with isoniazid. Of the two cases with initial PPD-positive results, one did not receive treatment and the other had treatment only irregularly. The rate of TB in screened patients was not greatly different from that of the background population rate: IRR 1.76 (95% CI 0.2–7.06) versus 12 (5.86–25.31) in patients who were screened inappropriately. In all, 1292 patients were treated with isoniazid, with 16 (1.2%) having increased LFT results that did not necessitate hospitalization or were fatal.

The experience of TB screening and infections in the ReAct trial with adalimumab is instructive [15]. Some 6610 patients were enrolled and followed for 12 weeks, with subsequent voluntary continuation for up to 5 years (median follow-up 211 days, maximum 669 days), representing 4210 patient-years of adalimumab exposure. This study was performed in Europe, which has higher background rates of TB and BCG immunization than North America. Indication for diagnosis and treatment of latent TB detected at screening followed national guidelines. Of the 6610 patients, 832 (12.6%) had a positive

Mantoux (PPD) test, and 196 (3.0%) had CXR indicating previous TB infection. Treatment for latent TB was initiated in 12.6% (835 patients). Twenty-one patients were reported to have developed TB during the study, confirmed by culture in 12, tissue staining in four, and not confirmed in five. Eleven cases were extrapulmonary. The median time to diagnosis was 6 months (range 1–14 months) after initiation of adalimumab. Screening results for these patients showed that eight had a Mantoux result of 5 mm or more in diameter. Isoniazid 300 mg daily was initiated in four of these patients, one patient stopping after 6 months as indicated in the local guidelines, suggesting resistance to isoniazid or non-compliance with therapy. The other four patients did not receive prophylactic therapy, because national guidelines used a Mantoux diameter of 10 mm as positive, or the patient had previously received BCG vaccination or recently stopped isoniazid after 11 months. One death was reported in a patient aged 86 years, who refused tuberculostatic therapy, with cause of death attributed to TB infection.

A similar result of screening has been reported from Japan, where 5000 patients receiving infliximab for RA were observed over a 5-year period. Fourteen patients (0.3%) developed TB. The initial rate of 0.6% in the first 1000 patients fell to 0.1% in the last 1000 patients enrolled, with a concomitant increase in use of isoniazid prophylaxis, rising from 13.5% to 25.5% of patients. Ten of the 14 patients who developed TB had CXR indicative of previous TB infection, with the CXR normal in two and not performed in two [34].

Surveillance of patients receiving TNF-blockers for reactivation of latent TB

Even in the setting of stringent screening, monitoring for TB during treatment is paramount. The above reports of comprehensive screening processes show that sometimes the skin tests and CXR are normal in patients who subsequently develop active TB. As the incidence of non-pulmonary TB is increased in this population, a continuing high level of awareness must be maintained. This continued awareness is emphasized by a report from Greece where screened patients developed active TB despite seemingly adequate anti-TB prophylaxis for 2 months before starting TNF-blockers [35].

Patients need clear instructions to report symptoms indicative of active TB. Normal features of active TB such as intermittent fevers, night sweats, cough and loss of weight may be present. Suspicion must also be high for lymphadenopathy, especially if isolated, and pyrexia of unknown origin. Minor CXR changes only, such as scattered small opacities on CXR or computed tomography (CT), can be seen in unwell patients who have miliary pulmonary TB. Some patients have few specific symptoms and suspicion should be high in a patient with a good response of the inflammatory disease to TNF-blocker treatment, but who has persistent malaise and 'failure to thrive'.

Opportunistic infections

Listeria monocytogenes infections have been reported at an increased rate [36], including septic arthritis [37]. *Listeria* is found most commonly in soft cheeses made from unpasteurized milk and in meat pâtés.

Less common serious infections have also been reported, including pneumocytosis and fungal infections such as histoplasmosis, aspergillosis, coccidioidomycosis and actinomycosis [38,39]. Areas in which histoplasmosis and coccidioidomycosis are endemic require consideration of the benefits and risks of therapy. *Candida* infections are almost exclusively of the mouth or oesophagus. The incidence of these infections is, however, rare. In the ReAct study [15], serious opportunistic infections (not including TB) were reported in 6 of 6610 patients: candida, 1; cytomegalovirus, 3; *Listeria monocytogenes*, 1; *Toxoplasma gondii*, 1.

Injection-site reactions

Injection-site reactions are the most common adverse event reported in clinical trials compared with placebo. Symptoms include erythema, localized pain and itching in patients receiving subcutaneous adalimumab and etanercept. They occur frequently in the first months of treatment, but usually resolve spontaneously despite continued treatment. The incidence in clinical trials was 40% for etanercept (placebo 13%) and 12% for adalimumab (placebo 5%). However, the number of patients who stopped treatment because of injection-site reactions was low (less than 2%). At times, the sites of previous injections can become inflamed at the same time as the most recent site injected. Recommended treatments consist of local cooling measures or antihistamine preparations.

Allergic, hypersensitivity reactions, anaphylactic responses

Allergic responses consisting primarily of localized skin erythema, itching and pain occur in about 12% of patients receiving subcutaneous adalimumab or etanercept. Anaphylactic responses have rarely been reported with these medications. Delayed hypersensitivity reactions have been reported uncommonly with all three drugs. Symptoms include myalgia, arthralgia, rash, fever, pruritus, oedema of face, lips, hands, dysphagia, urticaria, sore throat and headache.

These reactions are increased if there has been an interruption of the usual frequency of TNF-blocker therapy.

A recent report of skin abnormalities compared 289 patients with RA starting TNF-blocker therapy with 239 control patients not receiving TNF-blockers, matched for duration of RA disease [40]. The TNF-blocker therapy group took infliximab (167), adalimumab (108), etanercept (280), and lenercept (31), with a median follow-up of 2.3 years and a total of 911 patient-years. The TNF-blocker group reported 119 dermatological events in 74 patients: adalimumab 0.12, infliximab 0.14, etanercept 0.13, and lenercept 0.7 per patient-year. Nineteen patients stopped therapy because of the dermatological event. The most common skin events were skin infections (33), eczema (20) and drug-related eruptions (15); less frequent episodes were recorded of vasculitis, psoriasis, drug-induced systemic lupus erythematosus (SLE), dermatomyositis, and a lymphomatoid papulosis-like eruption.

Psoriasis

There have been reports of patients with RA, ankylosing spondylitis (AS), and Crohn's disease treated with TNF-blockers developing psoriasis or of worsening psoriasis in patients with psoriasis treated with TNF-blockers [41–43]. The mechanism may involve plasmacytoid dendritic cell precursors and type 1 interferon production [41].

Infusion reactions (infliximab)

Infusion reactions to infliximab in clinical trials have been reported in 20% of patients receiving infliximab, versus 10% in those receiving placebo infusions. About 3% of patients withdrew because of infusion reactions, and all recovered. The reactions usually consist of skin rashes, but malaise, abdominal discomfort, hypotension, and wheezing have been reported. Severe anaphylaxis including upper airway oedema, severe bronchospasm, and seizure have been reported rarely. Pretreatment with antihistamines, hydrocortisone, or paracetamol may reduce the incidence of infusion reactions. Infusion reactions are uncommon with the first infusion and increase after the second to fifth infusion; they may develop within minutes [44]. Reactions are sometimes preceded by feelings of non-specific malaise, and sometimes abdominal discomfort. Infusion reactions to infliximab are two to three times more common in patients who have developed anti-infliximab antibodies, and are probably mediated by these mechanisms. Infusion reactions are less common in patients receiving concomitant immunosuppresive therapy.

The treatment of infusion reactions depends on the severity of the reaction. Mild reactions are best treated by slowing the rate of infusion. Infusions must be given by staff trained in the management of anaphylaxis, with immediate access to appropriate drugs, including intramuscular adrenaline (epinephrine), intravenous antihistamine, intravenous corticosteroids, and artificial airways. It has been reported that pre-infliximab infusion of hydrocortisone or methylprednisolone can reduce the incidence of reactions [45].

Malignancy and lymphoproliferative conditions

The subject of the influence of new immunomodulatory drugs on cancer risk is very important but also very complicated. The background risk of different cancers varies in patients with chronic inflammatory conditions compared with the majority background population that does not have these conditions. Lymphoma is a good example of this. The incidence of lymphoma is increased with disease activity in RA to high levels in patients with persistent active RA [46]. In contrast, it is increased only slightly in Crohn's disease and psoriasis [47]. Comparisons with the general population probably do not reflect the true risk of different types of cancer in untreated patients with these conditions.

Clinical trial data and postmarketing databases have given conflicting data in patients receiving TNF-blockers compared with the general population for risks of lymphoma and some skin cancers. A meta-analysis of cancers diagnosed in patients in clinical trials of TNF-blockers reported an increased risk of skin cancers and lymphoma compared with that in patients receiving placebo therapy, but not compared with the general background population [48].

An initial report from the South Swedish Arthritis Treatment Group Register (SSATG) compared 757 patients with RA receiving etanercept or infliximab from February 1999 to December 2002 (1603 patient-years) with 800 patients receiving DMARD treatment from a community register followed from July 1997 (3948 patient-years) [49]. In the TNF-blocker-treated group, 16 tumours (five lymphomas) were recorded, compared with 60 (two lymphomas) in the comparison group. Comparison of patients with RA receiving TNF-blockers or non-biological immunosuppressive therapy with a background non-RA population gave a standardized incidence ratio of 1.1 (95% CI 0.6–1.8) and 1.4 (1.1–1.8) for all tumours, and 11.5 (3.7–26.9) and 1.3 (0.2–4.5) for lymphoma, respectively. The authors suggested that the increased incidence for lymphoma may relate to increased disease severity in those receiving TNF-blockers, and the increased incidence of total tumours in the non-biologic-treated RA population may relate to an increased incidence of smoking-related problems in this group. With regard to lymphoma risk, this study must be regarded as preliminary, owing to the low incidence of lymphoma in these patients.

Larger observational studies have given more information. Wolfe and Michaud reported results from a large longitudinal study of patients with RA followed from 1998 to 2005, with 19 951 participants encompassing 89 710 person-years of follow-up [5]. Of these, 68% received methotrexate and 55.3% received biologics. Ninety-five cases of lymphoma were identified giving an incidence rate of 105.9 per 100 000 person-years. Compared with the Surveillance, Epidemiology and End Results (SEER) database of the lymphoma rate in the background population, the standardized incidence ratio was 1.8 (95% CI 1.5–2.2). The odds ratio for lymphoma in patients receiving TNF-blockers compared with those not receiving them was 1.0 (95% CI 0.6–1.8), $P=0.875$). Methotrexate co-therapy with TNF-blockers did not change this risk. Infliximab and etanercept, which comprised nearly all of the TNF-blockers in this population, were not associated with a risk of lymphoma (adalimumab had just been licensed).

Wolfe and Michaud have also used this large observational database to investigate the risks of other cancers in patients with RA receiving biological therapy, mostly TNF-blockers, infliximab and etanercept (anakinra represented 2.5% of biological therapies used) [6]. They studied a slightly smaller population of 13 001 patients during 1998–2005, encompassing approximately 49 000 person-years, of whom 49% received biologics. They found 623 cases of non-melanoma skin cancer and 537 other cancers. Compared with the SEER database of cancer incidence in the background population, the standardized incidence ratios were: all cancers, 1.0 (95% CI 1.0–1.1); breast, 0.8 (0.6–0.9); colon, 0.5 (0.4–0.6); lung, 1.2 (1.0–1.4); and lymphoma, 1.7 (1.3–2.2). Biologics were associated with an increased risk of non-melanoma skin cancer (odds ratio 1.5 (95% CI 0.9–5.4)). No other malignancy was associated with biological therapy. These results were consistent across different biological therapies: infliximab, 33.1% (mean duration of therapy 2.9 (range 0.5–7.8) years); etanercept, 23.3% (2.7 (0.5–7.7) years); adalimumab, 5.9% (1.2 (0.5–7.7) years); and anakinra 2.5% (1.6 (0.5–3.9) years).

These results are in agreement with a report of another large observational study using a Swedish registry of patients with RA treated with TNF-blockers [50]. Askling *et al.* compared 4160 patients receiving TNF-blockers with 53 067 patients from an inpatient registry. They found the cancer risk for TNF-blocker-treated patients to be similar to that of other patients with RA who had not received these drugs.

However, in other inflammatory conditions with different treatment regimens, TNF-blockers may have a different outcome. In a group of patients with

Wegener's granulomatosis treated with etanercept, six malignancies were seen in the etanercept and cyclophosphamide-treated group compared with none in the placebo and cyclophosphamide-treated group [51].

Many chronic inflammatory diseases are associated with an increased risk of lymphoma. In contrast to the established risk of colorectal cancer in Crohn's disease and ulcerative colitis, the risk of haematological malignancies is marginally increased, if at all [47,52].

An increased association of haematological malignancies with anti-TNF agents has emerged as a cause for concern over the past few years [53,54]. Although the results from hospital- and population-based studies have conflicted, the results of a recent meta-analysis suggest that patients receiving purine analogues for inflammatory bowel disease (IBD) have a lymphoma risk approximately 4-fold higher than expected. Analyses of lymphoma risk in patients receiving biologic agents directed against TNF are confounded by concomitant use of immunosuppressive agents in most of these patients. Nevertheless, there may be a small but real risk of lymphoma associated with these therapies.

Recently, Biancone and colleagues published the results of a multicentre matched-pair study assessing the risk of cancer associated with infliximab. Some 404 patients with Crohn's disease treated with infliximab were matched to 404 patients who were infliximab naive. Nine of the patients with a history of infliximab use were diagnosed with neoplasia, compared with seven in the infliximab-naive group. The authors concluded that the frequency of newly diagnosed cancer in patients with Crohn's disease was comparable, regardless of their exposure to infliximab [55].

Hepatosplenic T-cell lymphoma (HSTCL) is an extremely rare form of non-Hodgkin's lymphoma, reported most commonly in adolescent and young adult males. The background incidence of HSTCL is unknown, because only about 150 documented cases have been published in the medical literature since it was first recognized as a distinct lymphoma subtype in the early 1990s. The clinical course of the disease is extremely aggressive, with a fatal outcome in most patients. Eight postmarketing cases of HSTCL have been reported in adolescent and young adult patients with Crohn's disease who were treated with infliximab [56]. The patients were all in the USA, ranged in age from 12 to 31 years, and had all received azathioprine or 6-mercaptopurine concomitantly with infliximab. In patients for whom the duration of infliximab use was reported, exposure ranged from one or two infusions to approximately 4 years of maintenance therapy. Three postmarketing reports of HSTCL have also been received in patients treated with adalimumab. Two were young men receiving Azathioprine or 6-mercaptopurine for inflammatory bowel disease [57].

A causative role for the TNF blockers versus combination immunosuppression in the development of HSTCL has not been established.

Currently this issue needs to be discussed with patients until longer-term data from the large longitudinal studies that include non-biologically treated patients with these conditions are available.

Drug-induced lupus-like reactions

Antinuclear (including anti-double-stranded DNA antibodies) and antiphospholipid autoantibodies are formed at increased rates in patients receiving TNF-blockers. In RA studies, positive results for antinuclear antibodies on at least one occasion were found with the following frequency: adalimumab, 12%, placebo 7%; etanercept 11%, placebo 5% (3% dsDNA/placebo 0%); infliximab 50%, placebo 20% (17% dsDNA/placebo 0%). It has been suggested that the rate of autoantibody formation may be higher with infliximab [58]. Although most patients do not develop clinical syndromes associated with these autoantibodies, all TNF-blockers have been associated with rare reports of lupus-like syndromes or antiphospholipid syndrome-like clinical scenarios, which resolved once TNF-blocker therapy was withdrawn. The lupus-like reactions consist primarily of skin rashes and serositis, with increased arthritis. The increased arthritis must be differentiated from secondary failure of the TNF-blocker with subsequent worsening of the original inflammatory arthritis. In the ReAct study of adalimumab in 6610 patients (median exposure 211 days), SLE was reported by investigators in two patients (0.03%).

Anti-drug antibodies (immunogenicity)

Infliximab, a chimaeric antibody, and certolizumab pegol, a humanized construct, contain mouse protein sequences (approximately 25% and 5% respectively). Adalimumab is a fully human IgG1 antibody that does not contain mouse protein sequences. Antibodies directed to all of the TNF-blockers have been detected in studies to date. Studies of infliximab and adalimumab have shown that patients who develop antibodies against these drugs may show less response to the drug and, in the case of infliximab, have more drug-related immune-mediated adverse reactions.

Clinical trials in RA demonstrated that approximately 5% of patients receiving adalimumab developed low-titre anti-adalimumab antibodies (AAAs) at least once during treatment (adalimumab package insert) [59,60]. Thus, adalimumab, like other TNF antagonists, may be immunogenic and can result in the development of AAAs. The rate of AAA development is reduced by concomitant methotrexate administration. Although there was no apparent correlation between the development of AAA and the occurrence of adverse events, these AAAs may reduce the efficacy of adalimumab. A report of 121 patients with RA followed for 28 weeks showed that AAAs were detected in 21 (17%) [61]. Patients with AAAs had significantly less improvement in disease activity, with a mean decrease in the disease activity score (DAS28) of −0.65 (SD 1.30) versus −1.7 (SD 1.35) for patients without AAAs ($P=0.001$). Patients who had AAAs less frequently took methotrexate (52%) than without AAAs (84%).

In 38 patients with AS treated with infliximab for 54 weeks (5 mg/kg on weeks 0, 2, and 6, and then every 6 weeks), 1 of 21 ASAS 20 (**As**sessment of **A**nkylosing **S**pondylitis Improvement Criteria) responders had detectable anti-infliximab antibodies, compared with 10 of 17 non-responders. Anti-infliximab antibodies correlated with lower trough infliximab levels, and infusion reactions occurred in six patients who were all antibody positive [62].

In a recent study, 61% of patients with Crohn's disease who received infliximab on an episodic basis developed antibodies to infliximab (ATIs), which contributed to a higher risk for infusion reactions and to a loss of response to treatment [63]. However, data from the ACCENT (**C**rohn's Disease **C**linical Trial **E**valuating Infliximab in a **N**ew Long-term **T**reatment) trials suggest that ATIs did not affect clinical responses and that either scheduled maintenance or concomitant immunomodulators reduced the incidence of ATIs [64].

In a phase II study, the cumulative incidence of antibodies to certolizumab pegol was 12.3% at 12 weeks in a cohort of 73 patients who had received three subcutaneous injections of certolizumab pegol 400 mg at 1-month intervals [65]. Although concentrations of certolizumab pegol were lower in patients who were positive for certolizumab antibodies, efficacy did not appear to be affected by antibody status: 44% of antibody-negative patients responded to treatment by week 12, as did 44% of the antibody-positive patients.

Studies of etanercept clinical trials have reported less than 5% of patients having non-neutralizing anti-etanercept antibodies on at least one occasion (etanercept package insert).

Congestive heart failure

Placebo-controlled studies of etanercept and infliximab in patients with severe congestive cardiac failure (CHF), New York Criteria grade II–IV, and left ventricular ejection fraction (LVEF) lower than 30–35%, demonstrated no improvement in outcome in patients receiving TNF-blockers, during the placebo-controlled phase. After TNF-blocker therapy finished, there was increased mortality in patients who had received infliximab 10 mg/kg, but not with lower doses. In the etanercept studies there was no significant increase in mortality, but a trend was noted in patients receiving etanercept [66,67].

Cases of new-onset CHF have been reported in patients receiving TNF-blockers, some of which resolved on stopping the TNF-blocker. In the ReAct study of adalimumab of 6610 patients (median exposure 211 days), 18 patients (0.3%) had CHF reported as a severe adverse event (SAE), 13 of whom had pre-existing cardiovascular disease excluding peripheral vascular disease [15]. In a recent report, although increased incidence rates of CCF were recorded in younger patients (age under 50 years) with RA and Crohn's disease, compared with patients not exposed to TNF-blockers, the numbers were so small with large confidence intervals that no adjustments could be made for pre-existing confounder status [68]. Of 4018 patients, 9 of 33 suspected cases were definite or possible.

The current advice is that TNF-blockers are contraindicated in patients with grade III–IV CHF and should be used with caution in patients with less severe CHF. Ischaemic heart disease without CHF is not a contraindication. A practical way to approach this scenario is to assess left ventricular output before beginning TNF-blockers, and to monitor this measure if adverse cardiovascular outcomes ensue. Other causes of these symptoms are many, including ischaemic heart disease and respiratory problems, including interstitial lung disease.

Neurological

A study of lenercept (a TNFRp55 receptor construct) in multiple sclerosis showing a worse outcome in patients receiving this drug [69], together with an early case report of infliximab [70], has led to the recognition that multiple sclerosis is a contraindication for TNF-blocking therapy. This has been reported for the three main TNF-blockers in use to date [71]. In the ReAct study of adalimumab in 6610 patients (median exposure 211 days), four patients experienced demyelinating disorders, all SAEs (0.06%): multiple sclerosis 1, central demyelination 1 (both confirmed by magnetic resonance imaging), Guillain–Barré syndrome (peripheral demyelination) 2.

TNF-blockers are therefore contraindicated in patients with multiple sclerosis or symptoms suggestive of a demyelinating neurological disease, the most common of which is transient loss of vision affecting one eye, suggestive of optic neuritis.

A recent literature review reported 15 cases of isolated optic neuritis occurring in patients receiving TNF-blockers, of whom eight had received infliximab, five etanercept, and two adalimumab. Eight patients had RA, three had juvenile idiopathaic arthritis, two had Crohn's disease, one juvenile spondyloarthritis and one psoriatic arthritis. All but two stopped TNF-blockers and all received pulsed intravenous steroids followed by oral steroids.

Nine patients had a complete resolution, two a partial resolution and four had continuing symptoms. Three patients with continuing symptoms had bilateral anterior optic neuritis, more suggestive of ischaemic or toxic pathology than of demyelination. The two patients who continued TNF-blockers had either partial resolution or continuing symptoms at 4 and 6 months [72].

Hepatobiliary

Isolated increases in liver enzymes, usually transaminases (alanine (ALT) or aspartate (AST) aminotransferase), have been reported for all of the TNF-blocker drugs. Very rare cases of jaundice and non-infectious hepatitis, sometimes similar to autoimmune hepatitis, have been noted. Very rare cases of liver failure have also been recorded, resulting in liver transplantation or death.

The frequency of LFT increases is more common in patients with AS, psoriasis and psoriatic arthritis, than in those with Crohn's disease, ulcerative colitis or RA, but has been reported for all indications. Most of these increases resolve with continuing therapy. In the IMPACT 2 (**I**nfliximab **M**ultinational **P**soriatic **A**rthritis **C**ontrolled **T**rial) study of infliximab treatment for psoriatic arthritis, more patients *not* taking methotrexate had abnormal LFT results than did those taking concomitant methotrexate [73]. In the EXPRESS (**E**uropean Infliximab for **P**soriasis [REMICADE®] **E**fficacy and **S**afety **S**tudy) study of infliximab treatment for plaque psoriasis, raised ALT/AST levels normalized in one-third of patients with cessation of treatment, in one-third with interruption of treatment and in one-third with continuation of treatment [74]. However, liver function must be monitored carefully as liver failure has been reported in patients receiving TNF-blockers. In some cases this SAE has occurred without significantly increased of liver function test results. No clear predictive signal for these rare SAEs has been identified to date.

Hepatitis B

TNF-blocker drugs are contraindicated in patients who are hepatitis B virus (HBV) carriers, as there is a risk of reactivation of hepatitis B infection. This is a similar situation to all other immunosuppressive therapies. A report of prospective hepatitis B and C testing before TNF-blocker therapy for Crohn's disease showed a deterioration of liver function in hepatitis B surface antigen (HbsAg)-positive patients [75]. In a recent case report [76], a known carrier with severe spondyloarthropathy already receiving methotrexate developed increased transaminase levels and HBV viral load after startinginfliximab. Liver function and viral load values normalized after treatment with lamivudine 100 mg daily while continuing infliximab once every 8 weeks.

The topic was reviewed in 2006 [77]. Current recommendations are that HBsAg-positive patients should receive prophylactic therapy with lamivudine or adefovir, as they are considered to be carriers of HBV with chronic infection. The area of uncertainty about prophylaxis surrounds patients who are HbsAg negative, as this usually indicates absence of ongoing infection. Successful treatment of a few HbsAg-negative patients with TNF-blockers without using prophylactic therapy has been reported [78]. The concerns are that rarely HbsAg-negative patients may be carriers and, on the other hand, that prolonged use of lamivudine can lead to resistant strains of HBV.

Hepatitis C

TNF-blocker drugs have been used in patients who are known hepatitis C carriers, with no reported worsening of liver function. Some reports show that LFT values have improved on therapy [79], including one report of a patient with both HIV and HCV [80]. Package inserts caution use in this situation.

Use in pregnancy

As with all new medications, caution in pregnancy must be exercised. All the TNF-blockers have been tested in animals and none has been found to have teratogenic potential. Several small series have recorded outcomes in patients who became pregnant while receiving TNF-blockers and were followed to the pregnancy outcome. To date there has been no recorded increase in adverse pregnancy outcome compared with that expected in the normal population. However, it must be emphasized that the studies to date are very small. These data are summarized in the very useful report from the Organization of Teratology Information Services (OTIS) Autoimmune Diseases in Pregnancy Project [81]. It is expected that adalimumab, etanercept and infliximab all cross the placenta similarly to normal human immunoglobulin. Pegylated products may not cross the placenta.

An abstract presented at the 2007 American College of Rheumatology meeting raised concern about the incidence of VACTERL congenital abnormalities, or components of this syndrome, from a search of adverse events for all three TNF-blockers reported to the US Food and Drug Administration (FDA) to December 2005 [82]. VACTERL is a non-random association of birth defects that occurs in approximately 1.6 in 10 000 live births. Mothers took a TNF-blocker at some point during the pregnancy. TNFβ (lymphotoxin-α), which is neutralized by etanercept, has an important role in the development of lymphoid tissue structure in developing animals, and lymphotoxin knockout mice have abnormal lymphoid tissue development [83].

There are no data concerning pregnancy outcome of fathers who were taking TNF-blockers at the time of conception.

Lactation

There are no reports of the effects of using TNF-blocker drugs in actively breastfeeding mothers. It is expected that low levels of drug would pass to the baby in breast milk, in a similar way to immunoglobulin, and infants do absorb immunoglobulins for the gut. A study of etanercept treatment (25 mg twice weekly) for a lactating mother with a postpartum flare of RA (who ceased breastfeeding) reported very low levels of etanercept in the breast milk [84]. The authors calculated that the daily amount of etanercept in breast milk would be 50–90 μg daily, giving a dose of 0.05–0.1 mg/kg. They state that the dose of etanercept for 4-year-old children is 0.4 mg/kg subcutaneously twice per week. Although a breastfed baby would receive a TNF-blocker orally, the activity of the drug is unknown and effects are theoretical.

Respiratory

In addition to the well documented upper and lower respiratory tract infections associated with TNF blockade, interstitial lung disease has been reported in patients receiving all TNF-blocker drugs [85,86]. These patients have usually had RA. Most forms of interstitial lung disease have been reported. Some reports demonstrate resolution of the condition on cessation of the TNF-blocker. A preliminary report from the BSRBR of a cluster of patients receiving TNF-blockers and azathioprine for RA showed a high mortality rate in a small number of patients receiving this combination of medications. A recent review of a large US database did not support this early report [87]. Most patients in clinical trials and postmarketing experience developing interstitial lung disease have been receiving methotrexate or no concomitant DMARD therapy.

Vaccinations

As with all other immunosuppressive medications, live vaccines are contraindicated in patients receiving TNF-blocker therapy. Commonly used live vaccines include the mumps component of many MMR (mumps, measles, rubella) vaccinations, oral polio (the intramuscular SALK vaccine is a killed virus), yellow fever, BCG, one type of oral typhoid vaccine (Ty21), and varicella [88].

Influenza vaccinations can be given safely to patients receiving TNF-blockers, with increases in antibody responses to the immunization, although these were significantly lower than the responses achieved in comparable healthy controls. A recent abstract of a placebo-controlled randomized study showed that the percentage response rate to influenza and pneumococcal vaccination in 99 patients with RA receiving adalimumab was maintained in comparison to that in 109 patients with RA receiving placebo injections. About 73% and 50% of patients in both groups without pre-existing antibodies developed antibodies to influenza or pneumococcus respectively [89].

A recent report in abstract form has suggested that patients with RA receiving etanercept ($n=12$) or etanercept with methotrexate ($n=7$) have significantly reduced responses to hepatitis B vaccination, compared with methotrexate alone ($n=4$). After 6 months, only 29–33% of patients responded, compared with 100% in those receiving methotrexate [90].

Use of TNF-blockers with other medications

The STAR (Safety Trial of Adalimumab in Rheumatoid Arthritis) and ReAct studies of adalimumab, and the ASPIRE (Active - controlled Study of Patients Receiving Infliximab for the treatment of Rheumatoid Arthritis of Early onset Study Group) study of infliximab, show that these TNF-blockers can be safely used with most other DMARDs. In RA it seems that there is at least an additive effect on efficacy of using methotrexate with TNF-blockers for all three TNF-blockers. This does not seem to be the case for psoriasis or psoriatic arthritis. The addition of etanercept and anakinra does not increase efficacy and is associated with an increase in infectious adverse events. Abatacept and TNF-blockers do not increase efficacy, but do have an increased of infectious adverse events.

There is limited evidence of the use of TNF-blockers with ciclosporin A, and no reliable evidence for cyclophosphamide or D-penicillamine. There have been no clear signals for interactions with any other medications.

Haematological

Pancytopenia has been reported with all three drugs. In the ReAct study of adalimumab in 6610 patients (median exposure 211 days), most haematological SAEs were unspecified or microcytic anaemia, with one case each of bone marrow suppression and pancytopenia; both patients received concomitant DMARDs [15].

Etanercept rarely causes neutropenia or pancytopenia [91].

Postmarketing safety experience in Crohn's disease

In 2004, Colombel and co-workers looked at the short- and long-term safety profile of infliximab in 500 patients at the Mayo Clinic [92]. The patients received a median of three infusions and had a mean follow-up of 17 months. Thirty patients experienced side effects in relation to infliximab, of which 3.8% were acute infusion reactions. The remainder consisted of serum sickness-like disease in 2.8%; three patients developed drug-induced lupus, and one developed a demyelinating disorder, with radiographic evidence of multiple sclerosis. Stopping the infliximab infusion resulted in partial symptomatic improvement, but no radiological improvement was reported.

Forty-eight patients had an infectious event, of which 15 patients had serious sequelae: two had fatal sepsis and eight had pneumonia, of which two cases were fatal. One of the patients developed candidal oesophagitis, one had severe viral gastroenteritis with dehydration requiring hospitalization, two had abdominal abscesses requiring surgery, and one had arm cellulitis.

Malignancy was also reported in nine patients. Two patients had a strong history of smoking, but were asymptomatic prior to taking infliximab. During therapy with infliximab, symptoms prompted a work-up revealing adenocarcinoma of the lung. Another 70-year-old patient was diagnosed with follicular non-Hodgkin's lymphoma within 5 years of initiation of infliximab. The rapid progression from previously documented pelvic adenopathy to lymphoma after infliximab therapy was instituted led to its implication in the process.

TREAT ([Crohn's] Therapy, Resource, Evaluation and Assessment Tool Registry) is a prospective patient registry that was established in response to an FDA mandate to study the long-term safety of infliximab in relation to other therapies for Crohn's disease. Patients participating in this registry reflect 'real world' experience, with 80% coming from community-based practices and 20% from university-based practices. Registry patients were treated using their own physicians' standards of care and were followed for at least 5 years. As of August 2005, 6273 patients had been enrolled of whom 3272 received infliximab (8314 patient-years) and 3001 received other therapies (6596 patient-years). Amongst the patients who received infliximab, 88% received at least two infusions. As of August 2005, the mean follow-up was 2.7 years. Patients treated with infliximab had, by definition, a higher use of other concomitant medications, and evidence of longer-standing disease; more patients receiving infliximab had moderate to severe or severe fulminate Crohn's disease, and had surgical or medical hospitalizations in the previous year. More patients were taking prednisone, immunomodulators or narcotic analgesics compared with those receiving other therapies ($P<0.001$ for all comparisons). As demonstrated by Cox proportional hazard analysis, treatment with infliximab was not associated with an increased risk of death or serious infection, although these were significantly higher in patients receiving prednisone or narcotic analgesics [12].

To clarify further the role of infliximab in Crohn's disease, an analytical decision model was constructed to evaluate risk versus benefit for this intervention.

A simulated analysis of 100 000 patients, divided into two arms (one receiving infliximab, the other standard therapy), showed that at the end of 1 year infliximab led to 12 210 more patients in remission, 4255 fewer operations and 33 fewer deaths. However, this was at the expense of an increased incidence of lymphoma (201 patients) and more deaths related to complications from infliximab (249 patients). [93].

The concern for the development of serious adverse effects to anti-TNFα agents, such as TB, lymphoma, CHF and demyelination, is fully warranted. However, it must be realized that patients with chronic inflammatory disease are already at an increased risk of developing these complications, as a sequela of their underlying chronic inflammatory state and/or concomitant use of immunosuppressive medications. Therefore, interpretations of the results of adverse events occurring in patients taking anti-TNF agents must correct for such baseline risk factors. Many clinical trials evaluating the safety of a new biologic are in themselves subject to fault. Limited sample size, different patient populations, the varying natural course of the disease and duration of study might overestimate or underestimate the true toxicity associated with the agent [94].

Given the tremendous efficacy that anti-TNF agents have had on the disease activity in inflammatory bowel disease, they should continue to be utilized safely in the short- and long-term management of Crohn's disease. However, close monitoring and efficient reporting of adverse effects should be encouraged. Developing an efficient multidisciplinary team composed of surgeon, infectious disease specialist and gastroenterologist will help to reduce the risks associated with these agents while maximizing benefits to the patient.

References

1 McCabe RP, Woody J, van Deventer SJ, *et al*. A multicenter trial of cA2 anti-TNF chimeric monoclonal antibody in patients with active Crohn's disease (abstract). *Gastroenterology* 1996; **110**(Suppl 4): A962.
2 Present DH, Rutgeerts P, Targan S, *et al*. Infliximab for the treatment of fistulas in patients with Crohn's disease. *N Engl J Med* 1999; **340**: 1398–405.
3 Sands BE, Anderson FH, Bernstein CN, *et al*. Infliximab maintenance therapy for fistulizing Crohn's disease. *N Engl J Med* 2004; **350**: 876–85.
4 Targan SR, Hanauer SB, van Deventer SJ, *et al*. A short-term study of chimeric monoclonal antibody cA2 to tumor necrosis factor alpha for Crohn's disease. Crohn's Disease cA2 Study Group. *N Engl J Med* 1997; **337**: 1029–35.
5 Wolfe F and Michaud K. The effect of methotrexate and anti-tumor necrosis factor therapy on the risk of lymphoma in rheumatoid arthritis in 19,562 patients during 89,710 person-years of observation. *Arthritis Rheum* 2007; **56**: 1433–9.

6. Wolfe F and Michaud K. Biologic treatment of rheumatoid arthritis and the risk of malignancy: analyses from a large US observational study. *Arthritis Rheum* 2007; **56**: 2886–95.
7. Westhovens R, Yocum D, Han J, et al. The safety of infliximab, combined with background treatments, among patients with rheumatoid arthritis and various comorbidities: a large, randomized, placebo-controlled trial. *Arthritis Rheum* 2006; **54**: 1075–86.
8. Jacobsson LTH, Turesson C, Nilsson J-A, et al. Treatment with TNF blockers and mortality risk in patients with rheumatoid arthritis. *Ann Rheum Dis* 2007; **66**: 670–5.
9. Schiff MH, Burmester GR, Kent JD, et al. Safety analyses of adalimumab (HUMIRA) in global clinical trials and US postmarketing surveillance of patients with rheumatoid arthritis. *Ann Rheum Dis* 2006; **65**: 889–94.
10. Dixon WG, Watson K, Lunt M, Hyrich KL, Silman AJ, and Symmons DP. Rates of serious infection, including site-specific and bacterial intracellular infection, in rheumatoid arthritis patients receiving anti-tumor necrosis factor therapy: results from the British Society for Rheumatology Biologics Register. *Arthritis Rheum* 2006; **54**: 2368–76.
11. Amano K. Pulmonary infections in patients with rheumatoid arthritis who have received anti-TNF therapy. *Intern Med* 2006; **45**: 991–2.
12. Lichtenstein GR, Feagan BG, Cohen RD, et al. Serious infections and mortality in association with therapies for Crohn's disease: TREAT registry. *Clin Gastroenterol Hepatol* 2006; **4**: 621–30.
13. Dixon WG, Symmons DP, Lunt M, Watson KD, Hyrich KL (British Society for Rheumatology Biologics Register Control Centre Consortium), and Silman AJ (British Society for Rheumatology Biologics Register). Serious infection following anti-tumor necrosis factor alpha therapy in patients with rheumatoid arthritis: lessons from interpreting data from observational studies. *Arthritis Rheum* 2007; **56**: 2896–904.
14. Kievit W, Creemers M, Fransen J, et al. A higher rate of serious infections in patients treated with TNF alpha blocking agents. *Arthritis Rheum* 2006; **54**(Suppl): S365 (Abstract 825).
15. Burmester GR, Mariette X, Montecucco C, et al. Adalimumab alone and in combination with disease-modifying antirheumatic drugs for the treatment of rheumatoid arthritis in clinical practice: the Research in Active Rheumatoid Arthritis (ReAct) trial. *Ann Rheum Dis* 2007; **66**: 732–9.
16. den Broeder AA, Creemers MC, Fransen J, et al. Risk factors for surgical site infections and other complications in elective surgery in patients with rheumatoid arthritis with special attention for anti-tumor necrosis factor: a large retrospective study. *J Rheumatol* 2007; **34**: 689–95.
17. Colombel JF, Loftus EV Jr, Tremaine WJ, et al. Early postoperative complications are not increased in patients with Crohn's disease treated perioperatively with infliximab or immunosuppressive therapy. *Am J Gastroenterol* 2004; **99**: 878–83.
18. Selvasekar CR, Cima RR, Larson DW, et al. Effect of infliximab on short-term complications in patients undergoing operation for chronic ulcerative colitis. *J Am Coll Surg* 2007; **204**: 956–62.
19. Centers for Disease Control and Prevention. Tuberculosis associated with blocking agents against tumor necrosis factor-alpha: California, 2002–2003. *MMWR Morb Mortal Wkly Rep* 2004; **53**: 683–6.

20. Bassard P, Kezouh A, and Suissa S. Antirheumatic drugs and the risk of tuberculosis. *Clin Infect Dis* 2006; **43**: 717–22.
21. Furst DE, Wallis R, Broder M, and Beenhouwer DO. Tumor necrosis factor antagonists: different kinetics and/or mechanisms of action may explain differences in the risk for developing granulomatous infection. *Semin Arthritis Rheum* 2006; **36**: 159–67.
22. Mohan AK, Cote TR, Block JA, Manadan AM, Siegel JN, and Braun MM. Tuberculosis following the use of etanercept, a tumor necrosis factor inhibitor. *Clin Infect Dis* 2004; **39**: 295–9.
23. Sichletidis L, Settas L, Spyratos D, et al. Tuberculosis following the use of etanercept, a tumor necrosis factor inhibitor. *Clin Infect Dis* 2004; **39**: 295–9.
24. Askling J, Fored CM, Brandt L, et al. Risk and case characteristics of tuberculosis in rheumatoid arthritis associated with tumor necrosis factor antagonists in Sweden. *Arthritis Rheum* 2005; **52**: 1986–92.
25. British Thoracic Society Standards of Care Committee. BTS recommendations for assessing risk and for managing *Mycobacterium tuberculosis* infection and disease in patients due to start anti-TNF-alpha treatment. *Thorax* 2005; **60**: 800–5.
26. Winthrop KL, Siegel JN, Jereb J, Taylor Z, and Iademarco MF. Tuberculosis associated with therapy against tumor necrosis factor alpha. *Arthritis Rheum* 2005; **52**: 2968–74.
27. Carmona L, Gomez-Reino JJ, Rodriguez-Valverde V, et al. Effectiveness of recommendations to prevent reactivation of latent tuberculosis infection in patients treated with tumor necrosis factor antagonists. *Arthritis Rheum* 2005; **52**: 1766–72.
28. Cunnane G, Doran M, and Bresnihan B. Infections and biological therapy in rheumatoid arthritis. *Best Pract Res Clin Rheumatol* 2003; **17**: 345–63.
29. Stas P, D'Hoore A, Van Assche G, et al. Miliary tuberculosis following infliximab therapy for Crohn disease: a case report and review of the literature. *Acta Gastroenterol Belg* 2006; **69**: 217–20.
30. Manadan AM, Poliyedath A, Sequeira W, and Block JA. Absence of transaminase elevation during concomitant methotrexate and isoniazid therapy. *Arthritis Rheum* 2007; **56**(Suppl): S171 (Abstract 316).
31. Mor A, Bingham CO, Kishimoto M, et al. Methotrexate combined with isoniazid therapy for latent tuberculosis is well tolerated in rheumatoid arthritis patients experience from an urban arthritis clinic. *Ann Rheum Dis* 2008; **67**: 462–5.
32. Ledingham J, Wilkinson C, and Deighton C. British Thoracic Society (BTS) recommendations for assessing risk and managing tuberculosis in patients due to start anti-TNF-α treatments. *Rheumatology (Oxford)* 2005; **44**: 1205–6.
33. Gomez-Reino J, Carmona L, Angel Descalzo M, Biobadaser Group. Risk of tuberculosis in patients treated with tumor necrosis factor antagonists due to incomplete prevention of reactivation of latent infection. *Arthritis Rheum* 2007; **57**: 756–61.
34. Dabbous O, Gilmer K, Tatsuki Y, et al. Tuberculosis in Japanese patients with rheumatoid arthritis treated with infliximab: findings from the Post-Marketing Surveillance Trial. *Arthritis Rheum* 2007; **56**(Suppl): S39 (Abstract CRC 13).
35. Sichletidis L, Settas L, Spyratos D, Chloros D, and Patakas D. Tuberculosis in patients receiving anti-TNF agents despite chemoprophylaxis. *Int J Tuberc Lung Dis* 2006; **10**: 1127–32.

36 Slifman NR, Gershon SK, Lee JH, Edwards ET, and Braun MM. *Listeria monocytogenes* infection as a complication of treatment with tumor necrosis factor alpha-neutralizing agents. *Arthritis Rheum* 2003; **48**: 319–24.

37 Schett G, Herak P, Graninger W, Smolen JS, and Aringer M. Listeria-associated arthritis in a patient undergoing etanercept therapy: case report and review of the literature. *J Clin Microbiol* 2005; **43**: 2537–41.

38 Jain VV, Evans T, and Peterson MW. Reactivation histoplasmosis after treatment with anti-tumor necrosis factor alpha in a patient from a nonendemic area. *Respir Med* 2006; **100**: 1291–3.

39 Bargstrom L, Yocum D, Tesser J, et al. Coccidiomycosis (Valley Fever) occurring during infliximab therapy. *Arthritis Rheum* 2004; **46**: s169.

40 Flendrie M, Vissers WH, Creemers MC, de Jong EM, van de Kerkhof PC, and van Riel PL. Dermatological conditions during TNF-alpha-blocking therapy in patients with rheumatoid arthritis: a prospective study. *Arthritis Res Ther* 2005; **7**: 666–76.

41 de Gannes GC, Ghoreishi M, Pope J, et al. Psoriasis and pustular dermatitis triggered by TNF-α inhibitors in patients with rheumatologic conditions. *Arch Dermatol* 2007; **143**: 223–31.

42 Richette P, Viguier M, Bachelez H, and Bardin T. Psoriasis induced by anti-tumor necrosis factor therapy: a class effect? *J Rheumatol* 2007; **34**: 438–9.

43 Cohen JD, Bournerias I, Buffard V, et al. Psoriasis induced by tumor necrosis factor-alpha antagonist therapy: a case series. *J Rheumatol* 2007; **34**: 380–5.

44 Lequerre T, Vittecoq O, Klemmer N, et al. Management of infusion reactions to infliximab in patients with rheumatoid arthritis or spondyloarthritis: experience from an immunotherapy unit of rheumatology. *J Rheumatol* 2006; **33**: 1307–14.

45 Augustsson J, Eksborg S, Ernestam S, Gullstrom E, and van Vollenhoven RF. Low-dose glucocorticoid therapy decreases risk for treatment-limiting infusion reaction to infliximab in patients with rheumatoid arthritis (RA). *Ann Rheum Dis* 2007; **66**: 1462–6.

46 Baecklund E, Ekbom A, Sparen P, Feltelius N, and Klareskog L. Disease activity and risk of lymphoma in patients with rheumatoid arthritis: nested case–control study. *BMJ* 1998; **317**: 180–1.

47 Askling J, Brandt L, Lapidus H, et al. Risk of haematopoietic cancer in patients with inflammatory bowel disease. *Gut* 2005; **54**: 617–22.

48 Bongartz T, Sutto AJ, Sweeting MJ, et al. Anti-TNF antibody therapy in rheumatoid arthritis and the risk of serious infections and malignancies: systematic review and meta-analysis of rare harmful effects in randomized controlled trials. *JAMA* 2006; **295**: 2275–85.

49 Geborek P, Bladstrom A, Turesson C, et al. Tumour necrosis factor blockers do not increase overall tumour risk in patients with rheumatoid arthritis, but may be associated with an increased risk of lymphomas. *Ann Rheum Dis* 2005; **64**: 699–703.

50 Askling J, Fored CM, Brandt L, et al. Risks of solid cancers in patients with rheumatoid arthritis and after treatment with tumour necrosis factor antagonists. *Ann Rheum Dis* 2005; **64**: 1421–6.

51 Stone JH, Holbrook JT, Marriott MA, et al. Solid malignancies among patients in the Wegener's Granulomatosis Etanercept Trial. *Arthritis Rheum* 2006; **54**: 1608–18.

52 Friedman S. Cancer in Crohn's disease. *Gastroenterol Clin North Am* 2006; **35**: 621–39.

53 Thayu M, et al. Hepatosplenic T-cell lymphoma in an adolescent patient after immunomodulator and biologic therapy for Crohn disease. *J Pediatr Gastroenterol Nutr* 2005; **40**: 220–2.
54 Losco A, Granelli U, Cassani B, et al. Epstein–Barr virus-associated lymphoma in Crohn's disease. *Inflamm Bowel Dis* 2004; **10**: 425–9.
55 Biancone L, Orlando A, Kohn A, et al. Infliximab and newly diagnosed neoplasia in Crohn's disease: a multicentre matched pair study. *Gut* 2006; **55**: 228–33.
56 Centocor. Press release. 22 May 2006.
57 Dear Healthcare Professional letter. Abbott, 16 July 2008.
58 Eriksson C, Engstrand S, Sundqvist KG, and Rantapaa-Dahlqvist S. Autoantibody formation in patients with rheumatoid arthritis treated with anti-TNF alpha. *Ann Rheum Dis* 2005; **64**: 403–7.
59 Adalimumab package insert. Chicago: Abbott Laboratories, 2006.
60 Hanauer SB, Sandborn WJ, Rutgeerts P, et al. Human anti-tumor necrosis factor monoclonal antibody (adalimumab) in Crohn's disease: the CLASSIC-I trial. *Gastroenterology* 2006; **130**: 323–33.
61 Bartelds GM, Wijbrandts CA, Nurmohamed MT, et al. Clinical response to adalimumab: relationship to anti-adalimumab antibodies and serum adalimumab concentrations in rheumatoid arthritis. *Ann Rheum Dis* 2007; **66**: 921–6.
62 de Vries M, Wolbink G, Stapel S, et al. Decreased clinical response to infliximab in ankylosing spondylitis is correlated to anti-infliximab formation. *Ann Rheum Dis* 2007; **66**: 1252–4.
63 Baert F, Noman M, Vermeire S, et al. Influence of immunogenicity on the long-term efficacy of infliximab in Crohn's disease. *N Engl J Med* 2003; **348**: 601–8.
64 Hanauer SB, Feagan BG, Lichtenstein GR, et al.; ACCENT I Study Group. Maintenance infliximab for Crohn's disease: the ACCENT I randomised trial. *Lancet* 2002; **359**: 1541–9.
65 Schreiber S, Rutgeerts P, Fedorak RN, et al.; CDP870 Crohn's Disease Study Group. A randomized, placebo-controlled trial of certolizumab pegol (CDP870) for treatment of Crohn's disease. *Gastroenterology* 2005; **129**: 807–18 [erratum in *Gastroenterology* 2005; **129**: 1808].
66 Khanna D, McMahon M, and Furst DE. Anti-tumor necrosis factor alpha therapy and heart failure: what have we learned and where do we go from here? *Arthritis Rheum* 2004; **50**: 1040–50.
67 Anker SD, Coats AJ. How to RECOVER from RENAISSANCE? The significance of the results of RECOVER, RENAISSANCE, RENEWAL and ATTACH. *Int J Cardiol* 2002; **86**: 123–30.
68 Curtis JR, Kramer JM, Martin C, et al. Heart failure amoung younger rheumatoid arthritis and Crohn's patients exposed to TNF-alpha antagonists. *Rheumatology (Oxford)* 2007; **46**: 1688–93.
69 The Lenercept Multiple Sclerosis Study Group and The University of British Columbia MS/MRI Analysis Group. TNF neutralization in MS: results of a randomized, placebo-controlled multicenter study. *Neurology* 1999; **53**: 444–5.
70 Van Oosten BW, Barkhoof F, Tryen L, et al. Increased MRI activity and immune activation in two patients with monoclonal anti-tumor necrosis factor antibody cA2. *Neurology* 1996; **47**: 1531.

71 Bensouda-Grimaldi L, Mulleman D, Valat JP, and Autret-Leca E. Adalimumab-associated multiple sclerosis. *J Rheumatol* 2007; **34**: 239–40.

72 Simsek I, Erdem H, Pay S, Sobaci G, and Dinc A. Optic neuritis occurring after anti-tumour necrosis factor a therapy. *Ann Rheum Dis* 2007; **66**: 1255–8.

73 Antoni C, Krueger G G, de Vlam K, *et al*. Infliximab improves signs and symptoms of psoriatic arthritis: results of the IMPACT 2 trial. *Ann Rheum Dis* 2005; **64**: 1150–7.

74 Reich K, Nestle FO, Papp K, *et al*.; EXPRESS Study Investigators. Infliximab induction and maintenance therapy for moderate-to-severe psoriasis: a phase III, multicentre, double-blind trial. *Lancet* 2005; **366**: 1367–74.

75 Esteve M, Saro C, Gonzalez-Huix F, Suarez F, Forne M, and Viver JM. Chronic hepatitis B reactivation following infliximab therapy in Crohn's disease patients: need for primary prophylaxis. *Gut* 2004; **53**: 1363–5.

76 Wendling D, Auge B, Bettinger D, *et al*. Reactivation of a latent precore mutant hepatitis B virus related chronic hepatitis during infliximab treatment for severe spondylarthropathy. *Ann Rheum Dis* 2005; **64**: 788–9.

77 Calabrese L, Zein N, and Vassilopoulos D. Hepatitis B virus (HBV) reactivation with immunosuppressive therapy in rheumatic diseases: assessment and preventive strategies. *Ann Rheum Dis* 2006; **65**: 983–9.

78 Raftery G, Griffiths B, Kay L, and Kane D. Chronic viral hepatitis and TNF- α blockade. *Rheumatology* 2007; **46**: 1381.

79 Khanna M, Shirodkar MA, Gottlieb AB. Etanercept therapy in patients with autoimmunity and hepatitis C. *J Dermatolog Treat* 2003; **14**: 229–32.

80 Linardaki G, Katsarou O, Ioannidou P, Karafoulidou A, and Boki K. Effective etanercept treatment for psoriatic arthritis complicating concomitant human immunodeficiency virus and hepatitis C virus infection. *J Rheumatol* 2007; **34**: 1353–5.

81 Chambers CD, Tutuncu ZN, Johnson D, and Jones KL. Human pregnancy safety for agents used to treat rheumatoid arthritis: adequacy of available information and strategies for developing post-marketing data. *Arthritis Res Ther* 2006; **8**: 215.

82 Carter JD, Ladhani A, Ricca L, Valeriano J, and Vasey F. A safety assessment of TNF antagonists during pregnancy: a review of the FDA database. *Arthritis Rheum* 2007; **56**: S41 (Abstract CRC20).

83 Davis IA, Knight KA, and Rouse BT. The spleen and organized lymph nodes are not essential for the development of gut-induced mucosal immune responses in lymphotoxin-alpha deficient mice. *Clin Immunol Immunopathol* 1998; **89**: 150–9.

84 Ostensen M and Eigenmann GO. Etanercept in breast milk. *J Rheumatol* 2004; **31**: 1017–18 (Letter).

85 Ostor AJ, Chilvers ER, Somerville MF, *et al*. Pulmonary complications of infliximab therapy in patients with rheumatoid arthritis. *J Rheumatol* 2006; **33**: 622–8.

86 Hagiwara K, Sato T, Takagi-Kobayashi S, Hasegawa S, Shigihara N, and Akiyama O. Acute exacerbation of preexisting interstitial lung disease after administration of etanercept for rheumatoid arthritis. *J Rheumatol* 2007; **34**: 1151–4.

87 Wolfe F, Caplan L, and Michaud K. Rheumatoid arthritis treatment and the risk of severe interstitial lung disease. *Scand J Rheumatol* 2007; **36**: 172–8.

88 Salisbury D, Ramsay M, Noakes K (eds) *Immunisation Against Diseases*. London: The Stationery Office, 2006.

89 Fomin I, Caspi D, Levy V, *et al*. Vaccination against influenza in rheumatoid arthritis: the effect of disease modifying drugs, including TNF alpha blockers. *Ann Rheum Dis* 2006; **65**: 191–4.

90 Ravikumar R, Owen T, Barnard J, *et al*. Anti-TNF therapy in RA patients alters hepatitis B vaccine responses. *Arthritis Rheum* 2006; **54**(Suppl): S366 (Abstract 827).

91 Kuruville J, Leitch HA, Vickers LM, *et al*. Aplastic anaemia following administration of a tumour necrosis factor-alpha inhibitor. *Eur J Haematol* 2003; **71**: 396–8.

92 Colombel JF, Loftus EV Jr, Tremaine WJ, *et al*. The safety profile of infliximab in patients with Crohn's disease: the Mayo Clinic experience in 500 patients. *Gastroenterology* 2004; **126**: 19–31.

93 Siegel CA, Hur C, Korzenik JR, *et al*. Risks and benefits of infliximab for the treatment of Crohn's disease. *Clin Gastroenterol Hepatol* 2006; **4**: 1017–24.

94 Hyrich KL. Assessing the safety of biologic therapies in rheumatoid arthritis: the challenges of study design. *J Rheumatol Suppl* 2005; **72**: 48–50.

2
Rheumatology

Rheumatoid arthritis

Rheumatoid arthritis (RA) is characterized by a highly variable outcome. The introduction of biological therapy for patients with active RA uncontrolled by conventional therapies used at appropriate doses has been a great advance. Many severe manifestations of the disease occur after an interval, making treatment choices in early RA an important clinical issue. Studies of tumour necrosis factor (TNF)-blocker therapies in early RA (duration less than 1 year) have made this an even more critical question.

TNF-blockers

Meta-analysis of studies in patients with RA show that there is little difference in the clinical and adverse effect profile of the three regularly used TNF-blocking drugs, adalimumab, etanercept, and infliximab [1–3]. The choice of which TNF-blocker to use for a specific patient will depend on more subtle factors not assessed in these types of analysis, on drug availability, and on the specific environment in which the drug is to be used. All three TNF-blocker therapies substantially reduce joint damage progression, improve patient well-being, and may increase return to work [4,5].

In early RA, patients treated with TNF-blockers in combination with methotrexate (MTX) have improved clinical and functional outcomes, and accumulate less joint damage than in patients treated with conventional MTX monotherapy or TNF-blocker monotherapy [6,7]. Two studies of infliximab use in very early RA have suggested that there is a long-term effect that allows the infliximab to be stopped in some patients, and the use of disease-modifying antirheumatic drugs (DMARDs), or in some cases no therapy, to maintain very good responses [8,9].

The BeSt (**Be**handel**St**rategieen voor Reumatoide Arthritis) Treatment Strategies for Rheumatoid Arthritis study compared four different treatment strategies in patients with early RA who had not received DMARD treatment. Patients who did not achieve the treatment goal of a Disease Activity Score (DAS) 44 <2.4 every 3 months had their treatment changed, following a specific protocol for each of the four strategy groups. Patients were randomized into one of the following groups:

1. Sequential DMARDs, beginning with MTX monotherapy 15 mg weekly escalated to 25–30 mg/week if the DAS44 was >2.4. (DAS44 ≤ 2.4 = low disease activity) Subsequent steps for patients not achieving DAS44 responses were sulfasalazine monotherapy, leflunomide monotherapy, MTX with infliximab, gold with methylprednisolone, and, finally, MTX with ciclosporin A and prednisone.

2. Combination therapy started with 15 mg/week MTX monotherapy increased to 25–30 mg/week if the DAS44 was >2.4. If response to therapy was insufficient, sulfasalazine was added, followed by the addition of hydroxychloroquine and then prednisone. Patients whose disease failed to respond to the combination of these four drugs then started MTX with infliximab, MTX with ciclosporin A and prednisone, and, finally, leflunomide.

3. The COBRA (combination therapy in rheumatoid arthritis) study step-down protocol, starting with a combination of 7.5 mg/week MTX, 2000 mg/day sulphasalazine, and 60 mg/day prednisone which was tapered to 7.5 mg/day over 7 weeks. If a DAS44 >2.4 was not achieved, MTX was increased to 25–30 mg/week; if the response was still insufficient, the combination was replaced subsequently by the combination of MTX ciclosporin A and prednisone, followed by MTX with infliximab, leflunomide monotherapy, gold with methylprednisolone, and, finally, azathioprine with prednisone. In good responders with a persistent DAS44 ≤ 2.4, prednisone was initially tapered to zero after 28 weeks, and then MTX was tapered to zero after 40 weeks.

4. Infliximab 3 mg/kg plus 25–30 mg MTX per week. After 3 months, the dose of infliximab was increased to 6 mg/kg every 8 weeks if the DAS44 was >2.4. Extra DAS44 calculations for dose adjustments were performed every 8 weeks within 1 week before the next infusion of infliximab. If the DAS44 was >2.4, the dose of the next infusion was increased to 7.5 mg/kg every 8 weeks and finally to 10 mg/kg every 8 weeks. If patients still had a DAS44 >2.4 while receiving MTX with 10 mg/kg infliximab, treatment was changed to sulfasalazine, then to leflunomide, then to the combination of MTX, ciclosporin A and prednisone, then to gold with methylprednisolone, and, finally, to azathioprine with prednisone. In good responders (DAS44 ≤2.4 for at least 6 months), the dose of infliximab was reduced (from 10 to 7.5, 6, and then 3 mg/kg) every next infusion until stopped.

The primary outcome measure was improvement in function assessed by the Dutch Health Assessment Questionnaire (D-HAQ). The study showed that beginning therapy with infliximab and MTX, or the COBRA protocol, gave superior results compared with monotherapy or combination therapy [10]. The protocol reported in the COBRA study of high-dose oral corticosteroids followed by step-down therapy showed similar clinical efficacy to infliximab and MTX, but had higher dropouts due to adverse events. Reduction of joint damage was impressive in groups 3 and 4. More patients in groups 3 and 4 than in groups 1 and 2 remained on their original treatments because of a sustained DAS44 ≤ 2.4: 48 (39%), 43 (37%), 94 (73%), and 102 (81%) patients in groups 1–4, respectively. Of these patients, 78% in group 3 had stopped prednisolone and 50% in group 4 had stopped infliximab because of a persistent DAS44 ≤ 2.4.

The 2-year follow-up data have been published, indicating that goal-directed therapy can achieve important clinical outcomes. These data include many patients now receiving infliximab who originally started in non-infliximab therapy groups. The overall percentage of patients in clinical remission increased from 31% after the first year to 42% after the second year. A total of 22%, 21%, 28%, and 40% of patients in groups 1 through 4 continued to achieve low disease activity score (DAS44 ≤ 2.4, 6 to 24 months).

BeSt	Treatment group	Low disease activity (DAS44 <2.4)	Mean improvement (D-HAQ)	Change in total Sharp score
Group 1	Sequential monotherapy (n=126)			
	3 months		0.4	
	12 months	53%	0.7	2.0
Group 2	Step-up combination therapy (n=126)			
	3 months		0.3	
	12 months	64%	0.7	2.5
Group 3	COBRA study protocol (n=133)			
	3 months		0.8	
	12 months	71%	0.9	1.0
Group 4	Initial combination with infliximab (n=128)			
	3 months		0.7	
	12 months	74%	0.9	0.5

These data are strongly supported by the PREMIER study (12 months) of adalimumab in patients with early RA with adverse prognostic indicators, either positive IgM rheumatoid factor, or at least one erosion in hand/foot joints [7].

Treatment	ACR 50	Remission (DAS28 <2.6)	Change in total Sharp score
MTX alone ($n=257$)	46%	28%	5.7
Adalimumab alone 40 mg e.o.w. ($n=274$)	41%	23%	3.0
MTX + adalimumab ($n=268$)	62%	43%	1.3

e.o.w., every other week; ACR 50, 50% improvement in symptoms according to American College of Rheumatology criteria.

The BeSt study protocol mandated that patients with sustained DAS44 <2.4 for 6 months treated with infliximab would stop infliximab therapy. About half of the patients treated with the infliximab from study start (group 4) were able to stop the drug at 12 months. Some went back on to therapy but others maintained the improvement on either MTX alone or no therapy [11]. After 3 years, more patients in group 4 (17%) had been able to taper infliximab and retain remission (DAS44 <1.6) compared with the other groups (10%, 5%, and 9% respectively in groups 1–3) [10]. These data raise the prospect of an induction regimen of infliximab and MTX as first therapy for early RA, with subsequent low-level therapy.

Reduction in joint damage progression

The suggestion from the ATTRACT (**A**nti - **TNF T**rial in **R**heumatoid **A**rthritis and **C**oncomitant **T**herapy) study that joint damage progression slows even in patients who do not exhibit a clinical response to therapy [12] has also been shown in adalimumab studies and in the TEMPO (**T**rial of **E**tanercept and **M**ethotrexate with Radiographic **P**atient **O**utcomes) study of etanercept and MTX [13]. Patients enrolled in the TEMPO study had slightly longer disease duration, most were MTX naive, and the baseline rate of joint damage progression was less than in other studies. In a post-study analysis, patients receiving MTX alone showed a strong relationship between clinical and radiological responses [14]. However, in the patients receiving etanercept monotherapy or etanercept and MTX, clinical responses for the groups did not correlate with radiological progression, which was reduced substantially in almost all patients.

Reduction of cardiovascular events

Several databases of postmarketing use of TNF-blockers have shown that the rate of cardiovascular events in patients receiving infliximab and etanercept, as well as MTX, is reduced compared with that in patients receiving other DMARDs [15,16]. Most databases do not have enough data on patients receiving adalimumab to make useful assessments.

Switching of TNF-blockers

This is an area with few controlled studies and many anecdotes. The failure of patients initially responding to a TNF-blocker has been termed secondary failure. This is thought to be due primarily to the development of blocking antibodies to the biologic. The alternative scenario of never responding to a TNF-blocker is termed primary failure. In RA, uncontrolled studies have shown that patients who develop secondary failure to infliximab can switch to either etanercept or adalimumab and achieve similar clinical responses as they achieved initially with infliximab [17–19].

Switching patients with primary failure has also been reported in uncontrolled studies to achieve clinical benefit [18]. The problem of results from uncontrolled switching producing positive results by artefactual mechanisms was emphasized in one report [20]. Although switching primary non-responders to the other type of TNF-blocker, for example from an antibody to etanercept, is hypothetically reasonable, registry data cannot verify this reason [21,22]. Registry studies show that most patients are maintained on the second TNF-blocker drug after switching [21,22]. Studies of switching to a third TNF-blocker are limited by small numbers, but the responses are often poor [22]. The alternative strategy is to increase the dose of drug. A blinded study of this has shown a response in RA disease activity to a dosage increase of infliximab in patients with both primary and secondary failure [23]. However, blinded data from the PREMIER study of adalimumab did not support this concept [7].

Combination biological therapy

A controlled study of etanercept and anakinra showed no additional clinical benefit and a significant increase in infectious adverse effects [24].

An add-on study of abatacept and TNF-blockers also showed little useful clinical benefit, and likewise a significant increase in infectious adverse events [25].

References

1 Hochberg MC, Tracy JK, Hawkins-Holt M, and Flores RH. Comparison of the efficacy of the tumour necrosis factor alpha blocking agents adalimumab, etanercept, and infliximab when added to methotrexate in patients with active rheumatoid arthritis. *Ann Rheum Dis* 2003; **62**(Suppl 2): ii13–16.
2 Hyrich KL, Symmons DP, Watson KD, and Silman AJ. Comparison of the response to infliximab or etanercept monotherapy with the response to cotherapy with methotrexate or another disease-modifying antirheumatic drug in patients with

rheumatoid arthritis: results from the British Society for Rheumatology Biologics Register. *Arthritis Rheum* 2006; **54**: 1786–94.

3 Nixon R, Bansback N, and Brennan A. The efficacy of inhibiting tumour necrosis factor α and interleukin 1 in patients with rheumatoid arthritis: a meta-analysis and adjusted indirect comparisons. *Rheumatology (Oxford)* 2007; **46**: 1140–7.

4 Kavanaugh A. Economic consequences of established rheumatoid arthritis and its treatment. *Best Pract Res Clin Rheumatol* 2007; **21**: 929–42.

5 Han C, Smolen J, Kavanaugh A, *et al.* The impact of infliximab treatment on quality of life in patients with inflammatory rheumatic diseases. *Arthritis Res Ther* 2007; **9**: R103.

6 St Clair EW, van der Heijde DM, Smolen JS, *et al.* Combination of infliximab and methotrexate therapy for early rheumatoid arthritis: a randomized, controlled trial. *Arthritis Rheum* 2004; **50**: 3432–43.

7 Breedveld FC, Weisman MH, Kavanaugh AF, *et al.* The PREMIER study: a multicenter, randomized, double-blind clinical trial of combination therapy with adalimumab plus methotrexate versus methotrexate alone or adalimumab alone in patients with early, aggressive rheumatoid arthritis who had not had previous methotrexate treatment. *Arthritis Rheum* 2006; **54**: 26–37.

8 Quinn MA, Conaghan PG, O'Connor PJ, *et al.* Very early treatment with infliximab in addition to methotrexate in early, poor-prognosis rheumatoid arthritis reduces magnetic resonance imaging evidence of synovitis and damage, with sustained benefit after infliximab withdrawal: results from a twelve-month randomized, double-blind, placebo-controlled trial. *Arthritis Rheum* 2005; **52**: 27–35.

9 Goekoop-Ruiterman YP, de Vries-Bouwstra JK, Allaart CF, *et al.* Clinical and radiographic outcomes of four different treatment strategies in patients with early rheumatoid arthritis (the BeSt study): a randomized, controlled trial. *Arthritis Rheum* 2005; **52**: 3381–90.

10 Allaart CF, Breedveld FC, and Dijkmans BA. Treatment of recent-onset rheumatoid arthritis: lessons from the BeSt study. *J Rheumatol Suppl* 2007; **80**: 25–33.

11 Goekoop-Ruiterman YP, de Vries-Bouwstra JK, Allaart CF, van Zeben D, *et al.* Comparison of treatment strategies in early rheumatoid arthritis: a randomized trial. *Ann Intern Med* 2007; **146**: 406–15.

12 Smolen JS, Han C, Bala M, *et al.* Evidence of radiographic benefit of treatment with infliximab plus methotrexate in rheumatoid arthritis patients who had no clinical improvement: a detailed subanalysis of data from the anti-tumor necrosis factor trial in rheumatoid arthritis with concomitant therapy study. *Arthritis Rheum* 2005; **52**: 1020–30.

13 Klareskog L, Van Der HD, de Jager JP, *et al.* Therapeutic effect of the combination of etanercept and methotrexate compared with each treatment alone in patients with rheumatoid arthritis: double-blind randomised controlled trial. *Lancet* 2004; **363**: 675–81.

14 Landewé R, van der Heijde D, Klareskog L, van Vollenhoven R, and Fatenejad S. Disconnect between inflammation and joint destruction after treatment with etanercept plus methotrexate: results from the trial of etanercept and methotrexate with radiographic and patient outcomes. *Arthritis Rheum* 2006; **54**: 3119–25.

15 Jacobsson L, Turesson TH, Nilsson C, *et al.* Treatment with TNF blockers and mortality risk in patients with rheumatoid arthritis. *Ann Rheum Dis* 2007; **66**: 670–5.

16 Dixon WG, Watson KD, Lunt M, Hyrich KL (British Society for Rheumatology Biologics Register Control Centre Consortium), **Silman AJ, Symmons DP** (British Society for Rheumatology Biologics Register). Reduction in the incidence of myocardial infarction in patients with rheumatoid arthritis who respond to anti-tumor necrosis factor alpha therapy: results from the British Society for Rheumatology Biologics Register. *Arthritis Rheum* 2007; **56**: 2905–12.

17 van Vollenhoven R, Harju A, Brannemark S, and Klareskog L. Treatment with infliximab (Remicade) when etanercept (Enbrel) has failed or vice versa: data from the STURE registry showing that switching tumour necrosis factor α blockers can make sense. *Ann Rheum Dis* 2003; **62**: 1195–8.

18 Cohen G, Courvoisier N, Cohen JD, Zaltni S, Sany J, and Combe B. The efficiency of switching from infliximab to etanercept and vice-versa in patients with rheumatoid arthritis. *Clin Exp Rheumatol* 2005; **23**: 795–800.

19 Bennett AN, Peterson P, Zain A, Grumley J, Panayi G, and Kirkham B. Adalimumab in clinical practice. Outcome in 70 rheumatoid arthritis patients, including comparison of patients with and without previous anti-TNF exposure. *Rheumatology (Oxford)* 2005; **44**: 1026–31.

20 van Vollenhoven RF, Brannemark S, and Klareskog L. Dose escalation of infliximab in clinical practice: improvements seen may be explained by a regression-like effect. *Ann Rheum Dis* 2004; **63**: 426–30.

21 Hyrich KL, Lunt M, Watson KD, Symmons DP, Silman AJ (British Society for Rheumatology Biologics Register). Outcomes after switching from one anti-tumor necrosis factor alpha agent to a second anti-tumor necrosis factor alpha agent in patients with rheumatoid arthritis: results from a large UK national cohort study. *Arthritis Rheum* 2007; **56**: 13–20.

22 Hjardem E, Østergaard M, Pødenphant J, *et al.* Do rheumatoid arthritis patients in clinical practice benefit from switching from infliximab to a second tumor necrosis factor alpha inhibitor? *Ann Rheum Dis* 2007; **66**: 1184–9.

23 Rahman MU, Strusberg I, Geusens P, *et al.* Double-blinded infliximab dose escalation in patients with rheumatoid arthritis. *Ann Rheum Dis* 2007; **66**: 1233–8.

24 Genovese MC, Cohen S, Moreland L, *et al.* Combination therapy with etanercept and anakinra in the treatment of patients with rheumatoid arthritis who have been treated unsuccessfully with methotrexate. *Arthritis Rheum* 2004; **50**: 1412–19.

25 Weinblatt M, Schiff M, Goldman A, *et al.* Selective costimulation modulation using abatacept in patients with active rheumatoid arthritis while receiving etanercept: a randomised clinical trial. *Ann Rheum Dis* 2007; **66**: 228–34.

B-cell depletion – rituximab

Rituximab improves the signs and symptoms of RA, improves function, and reduces progressive joint damage. It has been studied in patients with RA who have failed on DMARDs alone and also in those who failed both TNF-blocker drugs and DMARDs. In both groups, rituximab was shown to be superior to placebo, although the results in patients who had failed previous TNF-blocker therapy were less impressive. The reasons for this are unclear, but similar findings have occurred with abatacept. The effects of rituximab in early RA are as yet unknown.

The first infusion of rituximab is not an easy one to give, with a higher reported incidence of serious infusion reactions than for other biologics. The incidence of serious infusion reactions is substantially lower in RA studies than when used for lymphoma. This may in part be due to the lower numbers of cells that are lysed in RA. Once the first infusion has been given, the second of the two-infusion course is less likely to be associated with reactions. A gradual improvement in disease activity should occur, which can be difficult to ascertain, as it may take up to 3–4 months. Responses can last for up to 18 months after the initial infusions. The criteria for repeat treatments are usually based on clinical reactivation of disease, with a suggestion that increases in C-reactive protein (CRP) levels may be a useful sign of the need to repeat therapy. It has also been suggested that the time to recurrence of disease reactivation is similar after subsequent infusions, giving the treating doctor an important indication for the timing of further treatments. One question is whether rheumatoid factor (RF)-negative patients respond as well as RF-positive patients and/or anti-CCP antibody-positive subjects. Most patients enrolled in the studies of rituximab were RF positive. Subgroup analysis of larger studies suggests that patients negative for RF or anti-cyclic citrullinated peptide (CCP) antibodies do not respond as well as antibody—positive patients. However, the numbers of patients in these subgroups are very small (approximately 40), and the definitive data await studies with adequate numbers of patients tested for both RF and anti-CCP antibody status, who are selected for presence or absence of either of these antibodies.

Anakinra

The use of anakinra in RA has been less than that of TNF-blockers, owing to a combination of lower efficacy and patient convenience.

Other rheumatological conditions

Biologic therapies have been of great benefit in the treatment of RA, psoriatic arthritis, and ankylosing spondylitis. Their use is being explored in many other inflammatory and non-inflammatory conditions. A large number of uncontrolled and a smaller number of controlled studies have been reported. For rheumatological conditions, the best data source is the Annual Consensus Update on Biological Agents for the Treatment of Rheumatic Diseases. This consensus statement is updated annually and, in addition to mainstream therapy studies, contains a very detailed list of the reports of the use of biologic agents in any rheumatic condition [1]. The next section summarizes results concerning some of the more common conditions or those for which more definitive data are available.

Sjögren's syndrome

Biological therapies for Sjögren's syndrome are well reviewed in a recent publication [2]. TNF blockade was reported to be unsuccessful in two placebo-controlled studies [3,4]. In contrast, B-cell depletion therapy with rituximab has shown promise, originally in open-label studies [2]. A recently published randomized placebo-controlled study compared rituximab 1 g infusions versus placebo infusions in 17 patients with Sjögren's synodrome [5]. At 6 months there was a significant improvement from baseline in fatigue visual analogue scores in the rituximab-treated group ($P<0.001$) compared with those receiving placebo ($P=0.147$), as well as a difference in the social functioning score of the Short Form (SF)-36 at 6 months ($P=0.01$).

Vasculitis

Various types of vasculitis have been reported in many series, sometimes with positive [6], and sometimes negative [7] results. One controlled study of Wegener's granulomatosis with etanercept was unsuccessful, and showed an increased rate of solid tumours in those receiving etanercept who were also receiving cyclophosphamide compared with rates in patients receiving cyclophosphamide alone [8]. Controlled studies of infliximab therapy for giant cell arteritis (GCA) [9] and polymyalgia rheumatica [10] have shown no benefit, despite high levels of TNF being expressed in the inflamed arteries. In contrast, a small randomized placebo-controlled study of etanercept versus placebo in 17 patients with biopsy-proven GCA who had glucocorticoid side effects, showed a non-significant difference in the porportion of patients with glucocorticoid-free disease control (50% versus 22.2%), in patients receiving etanercept [11]. Patients receiving etanercept had a lower cumulative dose of glucocorticoid over the 6 months ($P=0.03$).

B-cell depletion therapy may have a role in the treatment of some vasculitides and many other autoimmune conditions, including dermato/polymyositis, autoimmune haemolytic anaemia, idiopathic thrombocytopenia purpura, and antiphospholipid syndrome, although studies to date are small and uncontrolled [1,6]. Systemic lupus erythematosus has been the subject of many reports, and controlled studies are under way [1].

Behçet's disease

Behçet's disease, both ocular and systemic features, has been treated successfully with both infliximab and adalimumab in open-label uncontrolled series [12–14].

Sarcoidosis

Pulmonary sarcoidosis has also been the subject of favourable reports from small uncontrolled series [15], but the results of a preliminary controlled study of infliximab (5 mg/kg) showed only small improvements in respiratory function in response to therapy [16].

Adult Still's disease and autoinflammatory syndromes

Adult Still's disease may respond to TNF-blocking therapy, although the response to interleukin-1 blockade with anakinra may be superior [17]. Anakinra has been used successfully in the treatment of adult-onset Still's syndrome [18]. However, it has shown most usefulness in the autoinflammatory conditions (sometimes called periodic fever syndromes) characterized by high levels of systemic inflammation such as Muckle–Wells syndrome, neonatal-onset multisystem inflammatory disease (NOMID), or Schnitzler's syndrome [19–23].

Gout

Recently anakinra has been reported to have good outcomes in treatment-resistant gout [24,25] and pseudo-gout [26].

References

1 Furst DE, Breedveld FC, Kalden JR, *et al.* Updated consensus statement on biological agents for the treatment of rheumatic diseases, 2007. *Ann Rheum Dis* 2007; **66**(Suppl 3): iii2–22.

2 Ramos-Casals M and Brito-Zerón P. Emerging biological therapies in primary Sjögren's syndrome. *Rheumatology (Oxford)* 2007; **46**: 1389–96.

3 Mariette X, Ravaud P, Steinfeld S, *et al.* Inefficacy of infliximab in primary Sjögren's syndrome: results of the randomized, controlled Trial of Remicade in Primary Sjögren's Syndrome (TRIPSS). *Arthritis Rheum* 2004; **50**: 1270–6.

4 Sankar V, Brennan MT, Kok MR, *et al.* Etanercept in Sjögren's syndrome: a twelve-week randomized, double-blind, placebo-controlled pilot clinical trial. *Arthritis Rheum* 2004; **50**: 2240–5.

5 Dass S, Bowman SJ, Vital EM, *et al.* Reduction of fatigue in Sjögren's syndrome with rituximab: results of a randomised, double-blind, placebo controlled pilot study. *Ann Rheum Dis* 2008 [Epub ahead of print].

6 Lamprecht P, Till A, Steinmann J, Aries PM, and Gross WL. Current state of biologicals in the management of systemic vasculitis. *Ann N Y Acad Sci* 2007; **1110**: 261–70.

7 Sangle SR, Hughes GR, and D'Cruz DP. Infliximab in patients with systemic vasculitis that is difficult to treat: poor outcome and significant adverse effects. *Ann Rheum Dis* 2007; **66**: 564–5.

8 Stone JH, Holbrook JT, Marriott MA, *et al.* Solid malignancies among patients in the Wegener's Granulomatosis Etanercept Trial. *Arthritis Rheum* 2006; **54**: 1608–18.

9 Hoffman GS, Cid MC, Rendt-Zagar KE, *et al.* Infliximab for maintenance of glucocorticosteroid-induced remission of giant cell arteritis: a randomized trial. *Ann Intern Med* 2007; **146**: 621–30.

10 Salvarani C, Macchioni P, Manzini C, et al. Infliximab plus prednisone or placebo plus prednisone for the initial treatment of polymyalgia rheumatica: a randomized trial. *Ann Intern Med* 2007; **146**: 631–9.

11 Martinez Taboada VM, Rodríguez-Valverde V, Carreño L, et al. A double-blind placebo controlled trial of etanercept in patients with giant cell arteritis and corticosteroid side effects. *Ann Rheum Dis* 2007 [Epub ahead of print].

12 Accorinti M, Pirraglia MP, Paroli MP, Priori R, Conti F, and Pivetti-Pezzi P. Infliximab treatment for ocular and extraocular manifestations of Behçet's disease. *Jpn J Ophthalmol* 2007; **51**: 191–6.

13 van Laar JA, Missotten T, van Daele PL, Jamnitski A, Baarsma GS, and van Hagen PM. Adalimumab: a new modality for Behçet's disease? *Ann Rheum Dis* 2007; **66**: 565–6.

14 Sfikakis PP, Markomichelakis NN, Alpsoy E, et al. Anti-TNF therapy in the management of Behçet's disease: review and basis for recommendations. *Rheumatology (Oxford)* 2007; **46**: 736–41.

15 Doty JD, Mazur JE, and Judson MA. Treatment of sarcoidosis with infliximab. *Chest* 2005; **127**: 1064–71.

16 Baughman RP, Drent M, Kavuru M, et al. Sarcoidosis Investigators. Infliximab therapy in patients with chronic sarcoidosis and pulmonary involvement. *Am J Respir Crit Care Med* 2006; **174**: 795–802.

17 Fautrel B, Sibilia J, Mariette X, Combe B; Club Rhumatismes et Inflammation. Tumour necrosis factor alpha blocking agents in refractory adult Still's disease: an observational study of 20 cases. *Ann Rheum Dis* 2005; **64**: 262–6.

18 Fitzgerald AA, Leclercq SA, Yan A, Homik JE, and Dinarello CA. Rapid responses to anakinra in patients with refractory adult-onset Still's disease. *Arthritis Rheum* 2005; **52**: 1794–803.

19 Hawkins P and Larchmann H. Interleukin-1-receptor antagonist in the Muckle Wells syndrome. *N Engl J Med* 2003; **348**: 2583–4.

20 Goldbach-Mansky R, Daily N, Canna S, et al. Neonatal-onset multisystem inflammatory disease responsive to interleukin-1B inhabition. *N Engl J Med* 2007; **355**: 581–92.

21 Lovell DJ, Bowyer SL, and Solinger AM. Interleukin-1 blockade by anakinra improves clinical symptoms in patients with neonatal-onset multisystem inflammatory disease. *Arthritis Rheum* 2005; **52**: 1283–6.

22 Leslie KS, Lachmann HJ, Bruning E, et al. Phenotype, genotype, and sustained response to anakinra in 22 patients with autoinflammatory disease associated with CIAS-1/NALP3 mutations. *Arch Dermatol* 2006; **142**: 1591–7.

23 de Koning HD, Bodar EJ, van der Meer JW, Simon A; Schnitzler Syndrome Study Group. Schnitzler syndrome: beyond the case reports: review and follow-up of 94 patients with an emphasis on prognosis and treatment. *Semin Arthritis Rheum* 2007; **37**: 137–48.

24 So A, De Smedt T, Revaz S, and Tschopp J. A pilot study of IL-1 inhibition by anakinra in acute gout. *Arthritis Res Ther* 2007; **9**: R28.

25 McGonagle D, Tan AL, Shankaranarayana S, Madden J, Emery P, and McDermott MF. Management of treatment resistant inflammation of acute on chronic tophaceous gout with anakinra. *Ann Rheum Dis* 2007; **66**: 1683–4.

26 McGonagle D, Tan AL, Madden J, Emery P, and McDermott MF. Successful treatment of resistant pseudogout with anakinra. *Arthritis Rheum* 2008; **58**: 631–3.

TNF-blocking therapy in ankylosing spondylitis and psoriatic arthritis

The term spondyloarthropathy (SpA) encompasses a number of individual diseases, including ankylosing spondylitis (AS), psoriatic arthritis (PsA), enteropathic arthritis (spondyloarthritis associated with inflammatory bowel disease), undifferentiated spondyloarthropathies, juvenile spondyloarthropathies, and reactive arthritis. These diseases are characterized by inflammatory arthritis affecting axial and peripheral joints as well as potential extra-articular inflammation in the skin, gastrointestinal tract, and other organs. As a group, they have an overall prevalence comparable to that of RA [1]. Although once considered to be relatively benign diseases, there is growing evidence, particularly in PsA and AS, that many patients have significant radiographic joint damage, functional impairment, reduced quality of life, and long-term work disability [2–4]. Although DMARDs may have modest effects in peripheral arthritis and some other aspects of disease, they have been shown to be ineffective for spinal disease in SpA [4].

The three currently available TNF inhibitors, etanercept, infliximab, and adalimumab, have been shown not only to significantly improve the signs and symptoms of SpA, but also to improve functional status and quality of life, and even to attenuate disease progression [5,6].

Ankylosing spondylitis

Clinical trial measurements

Assessment of efficacy has utilized composite criteria that include different aspects of disease. The early studies used the Bath Ankylosing Spondylitis Disease Activity Index (BASDAI). Functional ability was measured by the Bath Ankylosing Spondylitis Functional Index (BASFI), and mobility of the spine was measured by the Bath Ankylosing Spondylitis Metrology Index (BASMI). More recently, outcomes have also been assessed using the ASsessment in Ankylosing Spondylitis (ASAS) international working group response criteria. Given the substantial efficacy of the therapies under study, as well as the desire of clinicians to eliminate disease to the greatest extent possible, studies have also begun to assess higher levels of response, for example the 'partial remission' criteria, as defined by BASDAI, BASFI, and BASMI changes. In addition to clinical metrics, the effect of treatment on inflammation and structural damage has also been assessed using various imaging techniques [7–12].

Open-label reports initially suggested the potential efficacy of TNF blockade. These were followed by more stringent double-blind placebo-controlled randomized clinical trials of infliximab [13–19], etanercept [20–26], and most recently adalimumab [27,28]. These studies show that TNF-blockers induce substantial improvements in the signs and symptoms of AS, and are greatly superior to placebo treatment. All three agents produce comparable outcomes. A substantial minority of patients achieve extremely high levels of response, including partial remission. Clinical improvement can be seen as early as 2 weeks after the start of TNF-blocking therapy. Importantly, clinical efficacy can be maintained at a consistent level, with continued therapy through 2–3 years of treatment [15–17,24]. Treatment with TNF-blockers does not seem to induce immunological tolerance or long-term treatment-free remission in AS. Virtually all patients with AS flare upon discontinuation of therapy, with the mean time to flare reported to range from about 6 weeks with etanercept to 17.5 weeks with infliximab [18,21]. This suggests that continuous therapy with TNF-blockers will be necessary to maintain clinical benefit in patients with AS. Encouragingly, restarting therapy successfully reinduced significant clinical improvement in most patients.

Analysis of treated patients has also begun to identify the characteristics of patients who are most likely to benefit from TNF-blocker therapy. It is well documented that increased levels of acute-phase reactants are less common in AS than in RA. In studies of RA there has been a generally poor correlation between baseline increases in CRP or erythrocyte sedimentation rate (ESR) and response to TNF-blockers. In contrast, patients with AS and increased CRP or ESR tend to respond better to TNF-blocking therapy [15]. This is all the more striking given that changes in acute-phase reactants are not part of the response criteria in AS, as they are in RA. It has also been noted that patients with AS who have greater amounts of spinal inflammation on magnetic resonance imaging (MRI) may also have a greater response to TNF blockers [8]. Importantly, these observed correlations do not imply that patients without raised acute-phase reactants or spinal inflammation on MRI cannot respond to treatment.

In addition to improving the signs and symptoms of AS, TNF-blockers have been shown to improve the quality of life among treated patients [25]. There are also data suggesting that therapy may improve extra-articular inflammatory involvement in AS. In a systematic review that included data from controlled trials and open-label experience, it was observed that flares of anterior uveitis occurred less frequently under TNF inhibitor therapy (6.8 per 100 patient-years) compared with placebo (15.6 per 100 patient-years) [29]. A smaller study that followed patients with previous anterior uveitis who had started TNF-blocker therapy found a significant decrease in episodes in patients receiving antibody therapy compared with those receiving etanercept [30]. A similar divergence of recurrence of episodes of inflammatory bowel disease with significant reductions only in those receiving TNF-blocker antibodies was also reported in a small number of patients with SpA related to inflammatory bowel disease [31].

Perhaps the defining characteristic of AS is ankylosis of the spine; therefore, the 'holy grail' of therapeutic outcomes may be the prevention of progressive structural damage. The progression of AS can be quantified and tracked reliably by plain radiography. However, the relatively slow rate of change largely obviates the utility of this method for assessing structural effects of TNF-blockers. Given the clinical efficacy of these agents, it would now be unethical to allow patients to receive placebo treatment for the several years that would be required to detect important differences in radiographic progression related to effective treatment [7]. Therefore, there has been great interest in alternative imaging methods, particularly MRI. Not only is this technique able to detect changes in the spine and sacroiliac joints much earlier than conventional radiography, it can also be used to assess and quantify inflammation. Using MRI, treatment with TNF-blockers has been shown to attenuate spinal inflammation [8–12]. Although the suppression of inflammation was maintained through 2 years of treatment, it was not completely eliminated in most patients [8,12]. The extent to which suppression of inflammation on MRI correlates with attenuation of structural damage as measured by plain radiography remains to be elucidated.

Using evidence such as that reviewed above, international groups of rheumatologists have created treatment recommendations for AS, and also specifically for the use of TNF-blockers in AS [32–34]. Although a full recounting of these guidelines is beyond the scope of this review, it is worth noting that they try to account for factors such as disease activity, previous and concomitant therapy, and other patient characteristics at the start of treatment, and also call for continued evaluation of response during therapy. These guidelines are dynamic, and can be expected to evolve as newer information becomes available.

There are a number of unanswered questions and other considerations that will affect the optimal use of TNF inhibitors in patients with AS. From a clinical standpoint, it will be interesting to see whether there will be differential responses to this type of treatment in heterogeneous groups of patients with AS. In RA, greater levels of clinical response and prevention of joint damage have been observed when patients with earlier disease were treated with TNF inhibitors. Whether patients with AS with less damage might progress less with effective treatment remains to be defined. Similarly, the extent of response among patients with far advanced AS, and whether they can respond to TNF-blocker therapy, should be assessed.

Regarding mechanistic considerations, several clear, detailed studies have begun to elucidate the immunomodulatory effects of TNF inhibitors in AS [35,36]. Correlations between observed immunological changes and response to treatment or other key clinical measures could be important in optimizing therapy. Interestingly, disparate effects on certain *ex vivo* T-cell functions have been observed with different TNF inhibitors [37,38]. Any relevance of these observations to clinical use of the agents remains to be shown. However, it does raise the possibility that, despite comparable clinical efficacy seen to date, there may be some distinctions between the TNF macromolecules.

Regarding therapy, questions remain about the optimal treatment paradigm. In RA, the combination of MTX and a TNF-blocker is the 'gold standard' based on synergistic clinical efficacy [39]. In AS, because MTX is not effective for spinal disease, it has not been added routinely in combination with the TNF-blockers. However, given the potential for pharmacokinetic benefits with the monoclonal antibody TNF inhibitors, and the clinical synergy as noted in RA, it may be useful to assess more rigorously the utility of this combination in AS. As noted above, even with the impressive efficacy of TNF-blockers in AS, most patients can be found to have residual inflammation on MRI. Therefore, additional therapeutic paradigms should be explored in order to maximize efficacy and optimize outcomes. Finally, with a greater realization of work disability in patients with AS [3], and given the substantial clinical efficacy of the TNF blockers, the acquisition costs of the TNF blockers need to be assessed in clear pharmaco-economic analyses so that their true utility can be assessed [40].

References

1 Healy PJ and Helliwell PS. Classification of the spondyloarthropathies. *Curr Opin Rheumatol* 2005; **17**: 395–9.

2 Kane D, Stafford L, Bresniham B, and Fitzgerald D. A prospective, clinical and radiological study of early psoriatic arthritis: an early synovitis clinic experience. *Rheumatology* 2003; **42**: 1460–8.

3 Chorus AMJ, Miedema HS, Boonen A, and van der Linden Sj. Quality of life and work in patients with rheumatoid arthritis and ankylosing spondylitis of working age. *Ann Rheum Dis* 2003; **62**: 1178–84.

4 van Dendern JC, van der Paar DT, Nurmohamed MT, de Tyck YMMA, Dijkmans BAC, and van der Horst-Bruinsma IE. Double blind, randomized, placebo controlled study of leflunomide in the treatment of active ankylosing spondylitis. *Ann Rheum Dis* 2005; **64**: 1761–4.

5 Anandarajah A and Ritchlin CT. Treatment update on spondyloarthropathy. *Curr Opin Rheumatol* 2005; **17**: 247–256.

6 Davis JC Jr. Understanding the role of tumor necrosis factor inhibition in ankylosing spondylitis. *Semin Arthritis Rheum* 2004; **34**: 668–77.

7 Braun J and van der Heidje D. Imaging and scoring in ankylosing spondylitis. *Best Pract Res Clin Rheumatol* 2002; **16**: 573–604.

8 Sieper J, Baraliakos X, Listing J, *et al.* Persistent reduction of spinal inflammation as assessed by magnetic resonance imaging in patients with ankylosing spondylitis after 2 years of treatment with the anti-tumor necrosis factor agent infliximab. *Rheumatology* 2005; **44**: 1525–30.

9 Marzo-Ortega H, McGonagle D, Jarrett S, *et al.* Infliximab in combination with methotrexate in active ankylosing spondylitis: a clinical and imaging study. *Ann Rheum Dis* 2005; **64**: 1568–75.

10 Baraliakos X, Davis J, Tsuji W, *et al.* Magnetic resonance imaging examinations of the spine in patients with ankylosing spondylitis before and after therapy with the tumor necrosis factor α receptor fusion protein etanercept. *Arthritis Rheum* 2005; **52**: 1216–23.

11 Rudwaleit M, Baraliakos X, Listing J, *et al.* Magnetic resonance imaging of the spine and the sacroiliac joints in ankylosing spondylitis and undifferentiated spondyloarthritis during treatment with etanercept. *Ann Rheum Dis* 2005; **64**: 1305–10.

12 Baraliakos X, Brandt J, Listing J, *et al.* Outcome of patients with active ankylosing spondylitis after two years of therapy with etanercept: clinical and magnetic resonance imaging data. *Arthritis Rheum (Arthritis Care Res)* 2005; **53**: 856–63.

13 van den Bosch F, Kruithoff E, Baeton D, *et al.* Randomized double blind comparison of chimeric monoclonal antibody to tumor necrosis factor (infliximab) versus placebo in active spondyloarthropathy. *Arthritis Rheum* 2002; **46**: 755–65.

14 Braun J, Brandt J, Listing J, *et al.* Treatment of active ankylosing spondylitis with infliximab: a randomised controlled multicentre trial. *Lancet* 2002; **359**: 1187–93.

15 Braun J, Brandt J, Listing J, *et al.* Long-term efficacy and safety of infliximab in the treatment of ankylosing spondylitis: an open, observational, extension study of a three-month, randomized, placebo-controlled trial. *Arthritis Rheum* 2003; **48**: 2224–33.

16 Braun J, Brandt J, Listing J, *et al.* Two year maintenance of efficacy and safety of infliximab in the treatment of ankylosing spondylitis. *Ann Rheum Dis* 2005; **64**: 229–34.

17 Braun J, Baraliakos X, Brandt J, *et al.* Persistent clinical response to the anti-TNF-α antibody infliximab in patients with ankylosing spondylitis over 3 years. *Rheumatology* 2005; **44**: 670–6.

18 Baraliakos X, Listing J, Brandt J, *et al.* Clinical response to discontinuation of anti-TNF therapy in patients with ankylosing spondylitis after 3 years of continuous treatment with infliximab. *Arthritis Res Ther* 2005; **7**: 439–44.

19 van der Heijde D, Dijkmans B, Geusens P, *et al.* Efficacy and safety of infliximab in patients with ankylosing spondylitis. *Arthritis Rheum* 2005; **52**: 582–91.

20 Gorman JD, Sack KE, and Davis JC Jr. Treatment of ankylosing spondylitis by inhibition of tumor necrosis factor α. *N Engl J Med* 2002; **346**: 1349–56.

21 Brandt J, Khariouzov A, Listing J, *et al.* Six-month results of a double-blind, placebo-controlled trial of etanercept treatment in patients with active ankylosing spondylitis. *Arthritis Rheum* 2003; **48**: 1667–75.

22 Brandt J, Listing J, Haibel H, *et al.* Long-term efficacy and safety of etanercept after readministration in patients with active ankylosing spondylitis. *Rheumatology* 2005; **44**: 342–8.

23. Davis JC, van der Heijde D, Braun J, et al. Recombinant human tumor necrosisfactor receptor (etanercept) for treating ankylosing spondylitis: a randomized, controlled trial. *Arthritis Rheum* 2003; **48**: 3230–6.
24. Davis JC, Van der Heijde D, Braun J, et al. Sustained durability and tolerability of etanercept in ankylosing spondylitis for 96 weeks. *Ann Rheum Dis* 2005; **64**: 1557–62.
25. Davis JC, Van der Heijde D, Dougados M, et al. Reductions in health-related quality of life in patients with ankylosing spondylitis and improvements with etanercept therapy. *Arthritis Rheum* 2005; **53**: 494–501.
26. Calin A, Dijkmans BAC, Emery P, et al. Outcomes of a multicentre randomised clinical trial of etanercept to treat ankylosing spondylitis. *Ann Rheum Dis* 2004; **63**: 1594–600.
27. Davis J, Kivitz A, Schiff M, et al. Major clinical response and partial remission in ankylosing spondylitis subjects treated with adalimumab: the ATLAS trial. *Arthritis Rheum* 2005; **52**(Suppl 9): S208.
28. Van der Heijde D, Luo M, Matsumoto A, et al. Adalimumab improves health-related quality of life in patients with active ankylosing spondylitis: the ATLAS trial. *Arthritis Rheum* 2005; **52**(Suppl 9): S211.
29. Braun J, Baraliakos X, Listing J, and Sieper J. Decreased incidence of anterior uveitis in patients with ankylosing spondylitis treated with anti-tumor necrosis factor agents. *Arthritis Rheum* 2005; **52**: 2447–51.
30. Guignard S, Gossec L, Salliot C, et al. Efficacy of tumour necrosis factor blockers in reducing uveitis flares in patients with spondylarthropathy: a retrospective study. *Ann Rheum Dis* 2006; **65**: 1631–4.
31. Braun J, Baraliakos X, Listing J, et al. Differences in the incidence of flares or new onset of inflammatory bowel diseases in patients with ankylosing spondylitis exposed to therapy with anti-tumor necrosis factor alpha agents. *Arthritis Rheum* 2007; **57**: 639–47.
32. Braun J, Pham T, Sieper J, et al., for the ASAS working group. International ASAS consensus statement for the use of anti-tumor necrosis factor agents in patients with ankylosing spondylitis. *Ann Rheum Dis* 2003; **62**: 817–24.
33. Zochling J, van der Heijde D, Burgos-Vargas R, et al.; 'ASsessment in AS' international working group; European League Against Rheumatism. ASAS/EULAR recommendations for the management of ankylosing spondylitis. *Ann Rheum Dis* 2006; **65**: 442–52.
34. Zochling J, van der Heijde D, Dougados M, and Braun J. Current evidence for the management of ankylosing spondylitis: a systematic literature review for the ASAS/EULAR management recommendations in ankylosing spondylitis. *Ann Rheum Dis* 2006; **65**: 423–32.
35. Kruithof E, Baeten D, van den Bosch F, Mielants H, Veys EM, and De Keyser F. Histological evidence that infliximab treatment leads to downregulation of inflammation and tissue remodelling of the synovial membrane in spondyloarthropathy. *Ann Rheum Dis* 2005; **64**: 529–36.
36. Kruithof E, De Rycke L, Roth J, et al. Immunomodulatory effects of etanercept on peripheral joint synovitis in the spondyloarthropathies. *Arthritis Rheum* 2005; **52**: 3898–909.
37. Zou JX, Rudwaleit M, Brandt J, Thiel A, Braun J, and Sieper J. Upregulation of the production of tumor necrosis factor α and interferon β by T cells in ankylosing spondylitis during treatment with etanercept. *Ann Rheum Dis* 2003; **62**: 561–4.

38 Zou JX, Rudwaleit M, Brandt J, Thiel A, Braun J, and Sieper J. Down-regulation of the nonspecific and antigen-specific T cell cytokine response in ankylosing spondylitis during treatment with infliximab. *Arthritis Rheum* 2003; **48**: 780–90.
39 Kavanaugh A, Cohen S, and Cush J. The evolving use of TNF inhibitors in rheumatoid arthritis. *J Rheumatol* 2004; **31**: 1881–4.
40 Kavanaugh A. The pharmacoeconomics of newer therapeutics for rheumatic diseases. *Rheum Dis Clin North Am* 2006; **32**: 45–56, viii.

Psoriatic arthritis

The treatment of patients with PsA requires consideration of the various potential areas of disease involvement, including peripheral arthritis, axial arthritis, skin and nail involvement, dactylitis, and enthesitis [1]. Although seemingly simple, in the clinic this represents a challenge, as all of the heterogeneous areas of involvement can vary from minimally involved to severely involved in a single patient. TNF-blocking therapy has proven effective in controlling inflammation in all of these distinct sites. The introduction of TNF-blockers has generated interest in defining and validating appropriate outcomes for varied disease manifestations in PsA [2]. There has been a progression in studies of TNF-blockers in PsA, with early open-label trials being followed by large randomized controlled trials [3–10].

Several important conclusions can be derived from these studies. TNF-blockers reproducibly induce substantial improvements in the signs and symptoms of peripheral arthritis in PsA, greatly superior to those with placebo. Placebo responses among patients with PsA generally seem to be lower than those in comparable studies of RA. The extent of response as regards peripheral arthritis appears comparable among all three TNF inhibitors. With treatment, a substantial minority of patients achieve extremely high levels of response, for example ACR 70 (70% improvement in symptoms according to American College of Rheumatology criteria). Clinical improvement can be seen as early as 2 weeks after the start of TNF-blocker therapy, and can be maintained, at a consistent level, with continued therapy through several years of treatment [5,6].

In addition to improving the signs and symptoms of peripheral arthritis, TNF-blocking therapy also improved functional status and quality of life [3–10]. Moreover, in several studies in which they were assessed, improvements in dactylitis and enthesitis were also observed [5,6]. Notably, treatment with TNF-blockers has also been shown to attenuate the progression of radiographic joint damage in the peripheral joints of patients with PsA [7,8,10]. Although PsA clearly has radiographic characteristics distinct from those seen in RA, such as proliferative lesions and gross osteolysis, scoring systems slightly modified from the standards used in RA (i.e. the van der Heijde–Sharp score) have been used in the studies, and have proven workable. Most patients do not have significant changes in radiographic scores during the course of the studies. Thus, overall differences in radiographic progression are driven by changes in approximately a third of patients with PsA. This has been accentuated by the need for radiographic assessments at shorter time intervals. With the proven efficacy of TNF-blockers, placebo treatment phases of longer than a few months are no longer ethical. Interestingly, a short placebo period (e.g. 4 months) followed by 8 months of TNF-blocker therapy has been shown to blur distinctions between groups [7]. This suggests that radiographic changes in PsA may be more plastic than those in RA, and highlights the need to assess radiographic outcomes at short-term intervals, such as 6 months.

Dermatological involvement is critically important in PsA, and skin responses to TNF-blocker therapy have been included in all PsA trials. Interestingly, although the extent of improvement in peripheral arthritis was comparable among agents, the extent of skin improvement appears to be greater with the monoclonal antibodies than with the soluble receptor construct. Whether this difference relates to differential mechanisms, dosages used (etanercept 25 mg b.i.w.; infliximab 5 mg/kg at weeks 0, 2, and 6 then every 8 weeks; adalimumab 40 mg q.o.w.), or some other factor remains to be defined. Interestingly, preliminary analysis of individual patient responses shows that there may be discordance between dermatological and articular outcomes in individual patients.

In studies of all three agents, concomitant stable use of MTX was allowed but not required. The concomitant use of MTX used by about half of the patients did not seem to affect any of the clinical or radiographic responses. Of note, this does not imply that this combination is not synergistic in PsA as it is in RA; to determine this, a study employing *de novo* initiation of all three arms (MTX, TNF inhibitor, MTX + TNF inhibitor) would be required.

There are still a number of unanswered questions surrounding the optimal use of TNF-blockers in patients with PsA. Analysis of treated patients to identify the characteristics of patients most likely to benefit from TNF inhibitor therapy would help refine treatment. Questions remain regarding correlations between the disparate outcomes of PsA and how each responds to specific therapies. Whether or not synergistic efficacy will be observed with the combination of MTX and TNF-blockers needs to be assessed. The potential for different responses among different subsets of patients, such as those with early disease, remains to be defined. Finally, with a greater realization of work disability in patients with PsA, and given the substantial clinical efficacy of the TNF-blockers, the acquisition costs of the TNF-blockers need to be assessed in clear pharmaco-economic analyses so that their true utility can be assessed [11].

Safety

Because TNF inhibitors have not had the same postmarketing exposure among patients with SpA as they have had in RA, fuller assessment of their real safety in the clinic and in more heterogeneous populations of patients than those typically enrolled in trials is eagerly expected over the next few years. Adverse effects already observed among the one million patients with RA and Crohn's disease who have received TNF-blockers over the past decade have been observed in patients with PsA and AS.

There are several factors that can be expected to impact the safety of TNF inhibitors in SpA in comparison with other conditions. First, because their introduction follows the experience in other conditions, patients benefit by the approaches to stratification and screening that have already proven useful, such as screening patients for latent tuberculosis prior to therapy. Second, in comparison with patients with RA, those with AS and PsA tend to be younger and to have less co-morbidity, which may be expected to decrease the incidence of some side effects, such as infection. On the other hand, some adverse effects, such as abnormalities in liver function, may be seen more commonly among patients with PsA compared with those with RA [12]. Patients with PsA who have been exposed to ultraviolet light therapies for skin disease may also have an increased risk of skin cancer.

References

1 Kavanaugh A and Cassell S. Outcome measures in psoriatic arthritis. *Curr Rheumatol Rep* 2005; **7**: 195–200.
2 Kavanaugh AF, Ritchlin CT; GRAPPA Treatment Guideline Committee. Systematic review of treatments for psoriatic arthritis: an evidence based approach and basis for treatment guidelines. *J Rheumatol* 2006; **33**: 1417–21.
3 Mease PJ, Goffe BS, Metz J, *et al*. Etanercept in the treatment of psoriatic arthritis and psoriasis: a randomised trial. *Lancet* 2000; **356**: 385–90.
4 Mease PJ, Kivitz AJ, Burch FX, *et al*. Etanercept treatment of psoriatic arthritis: safety, efficacy, and effect on disease progression. *Arthritis Rheum* 2004; **50**: 2264–72.
5 Antoni CE, Kavanaugh A, Kirkham B, *et al*. Sustained benefits of infliximab therapy for dermatologic and articular manifestations of psoriatic arthritis: results from the infliximab multinational psoriatic arthritis controlled trial (IMPACT). *Arthritis Rheum* 2005; **52**: 1227–36.
6 Antoni C, Krueger G G, de Vlam K, *et al*. Infliximab improves signs and symptoms of psoriatic arthritis: results of the IMPACT 2 trial. *Ann Rheum Dis* 2005; **64**: 1150–7.
7 Kavanaugh A, Antoni CE, Gladman D, *et al*. The Infliximab Multinational Psoriatic Arthritis Controlled Trial (IMPACT): results of radiographic analyses after 1 year. *Ann Rheum Dis* 2006; **65**: 1038–43.
8 van der Heijde D, Kavanaugh A, Gladman DD, *et al*. Infliximab inhibits progression of radiographic damage in patients with active psoriatic arthritis through one year of

treatment: results from the induction and maintenance psoriatic arthritis clinical trial 2. *Arthritis Rheum* 2007; **56**: 2698–707.

9   Kavanaugh A, Antoni C, Krueger GG, *et al*. Infliximab improves health related quality of life and physical function in patients with psoriatic arthritis. *Ann Rheum Dis* 2006; **65**: 471–7.

10 Mease PJ, Gladman DD, Ritchlin CT, *et al*. Adalimumab for the treatment of patients with moderately to severely active psoriatic arthritis: result of a double-blind, randomized, placebo-controlled trial. *Arthritis Rheum* 2005; **52**: 3279–89.

11 Kavanaugh A, Antoni C, Mease P, *et al*. Effect of infliximab therapy on employment, time lost from work, and productivity in patients with psoriatic arthritis. *J Rheumatol* 2006; **33**: 2254–9.

12 Cassell S, Tutuncu Z, Kremer J, *et al*. Psoriatic arthritis patients have different rates of adverse events than rheumatoid arthritis patients when treated with TNF inhihitors: analysis from CORRONA Database. *Arthritis Rheum* 2005; **52**(Suppl 9): S211.

Adalimumab (Humira)

Chemical properties	Recombinant human IgG1 monoclonal antibody, 148 kDa
Manufacture	Produced in Chinese Hamster Ovary cells
Stability	Stable for at least 24 months if stored in the dark at 2–8°C
Pharmacokinetics	After a single 40-mg subcutaneous injection, average peak serum concentration was 4.7 μg/ml after 5.4 days. Average bioavailability compared to intravenous dosing is 64%. Half-life is 10–20 days. Clearance in patients with moderate to severe psoriasis is probably lower than in RA studies
Metabolism	Unclear but thought to be catabolized in a similar manner to normal human immunoglobulin. In patients receiving adalimumab monotherapy, clearance in patients with RA is faster than in those with moderate to severe psoriasis
Drug interactions	Methotrexate probably decreases the clearance rate of adalimumab, although this does not depend on the dose of MTX (tested range 5–30 mg). Adalimumab does not alter MTX concentrations

Clinical trial data – rheumatoid arthritis

Phase I studies investigated intravenous adalimumab in doses ranging from 0.5 to 10 mg/kg. Subsequent studies using subcutaneous 0.3–1.0 mg/kg injections showed equal efficacy.

Phase II/III studies

The main outcomes measures for these studies were the American College of Rheumatology response criteria (ACR 20/50/70) denoting an improvement of at least 20%, 50%, or 70% in RA activity. These studies were performed in the USA, Europe, and Australia, and are summarized below.

ARMADA (DE009) – USA, Phase II/III [1] Patients not responding to MTX, average dose in active therapy group 16.8 mg, placebo group 16.5 mg per week. Mean age 55 years, 77% female, disease duration 12.7 years.

ARMADA	Dose (*n*)	ACR 20	ACR 50	ACR 70
	20 mg e.o.w. (67)	48%*	33%	10%
	40 mg e.o.w. (63)	67%*	54%*	24%*
	80 mg e.o.w. (66)	66%*	41%*	19%*
	Placebo (60)	13%	7%	3%

e.o.w., every other week; *$P<0.05$ vs placebo.

DE011 – Europe, Australia, Canada, Phase III [2] Adalimumab monotherapy, all patients previously received DMARDs. Mean age 53 years, 77% female.

DE011	Dose (*n*)	ACR 20	ACR 50	ACR 70
	20 mg e.o.w. (106)	36%*	20%*	9%*
	20 mg weekly (112)	39%*	21%*	10%*
	40 mg e.o.w. (113)	46%*	22%*	12%*
	40 mg weekly (103)	53%*	35%*	18%*
	Placebo (110)	19%	8%	2%

e.o.w., every other week; *$P<0.05$ vs placebo.

DE019 – USA, Canada, Phase III [3] Patients not responding to MTX, average dose in active therapy group 16.3 mg, placebo group 16.7 mg per week. Mean age 57 years, 70% female, disease duration 11 years.

DE019 Dose (*n*)	ACR 20 (week 24/52)	ACR 50 (week 24/52)	ACR 70 (week 24/52)	Change in HAQ	Change in total Sharp score (week 24/52)
20 mg weekly (212)	61%*/55%*	42%*/38%*	18%*/21%*	–0.60*	0.6/0.8*
40 mg e.o.w. (207)	63%*/59%*	39%*/42%*	21%*/23%*	–0.56*	0.3/0.1*
Placebo (200)	30%/24%	10%/10%	3%/5%	–0.24	1.3/2.7

e.o.w., every other week; *$P<0.001$ adalimumab groups vs placebo.

PREMIER (DE013) – Early RA – USA, Europe, Canada, Australia [4] No previous MTX exposure, either RF positive or at least one erosion on radiography. Mean age 52 years, female 75%, mean disease duration 0.7 years. Outcomes at week 52, remission defined by Disease Activity Score (DAS28) <2.6.

PREMIER	Treatment (**n**)	ACR 50	Remission	Change in Sharp score
	MTX alone (257)	46%	28%	5.7
	Adalimumab alone 40 mg e.o.w. (274)	41%	23%	3.0
	Methotrexate + adalimumab (268)	62%*	43%†	1.3‡

*$P < 0.022$ vs MTX alone; $P < 0.001$ vs adalimumab alone.
†$P < 0.001$ vs MTX alone and adalimumab alone.
‡$P < 0.001$ vs MTX alone; $P < 0.002$ vs adalimumab alone.

The PREMIER study protocol included a study of dose adjustment of the injectable treatment (adalimumab or placebo) to once weekly in patients who did not achieve ACR 20 responses on two consecutive visits after week 16. This strategy did not yield additional clinical benefit.

PREMIER: injectable dose increases	Treatment	ACR 20	ACR 50	Remission
	MTX (placebo injections)			
	Year 1	4%	1%	0%
	Year 2	4%	2%	1%
	Adalimumab (adalimumab injections)			
	Year 1	2%	1%	0%
	Year 2	3%	0%	0%
	MTX/adalimumab (adalimumab injections)			
	Year 1	1%	1%	1%
	Year 2	1%	1%	1%

STAR (DE031) – USA, Phase III [5] Adalimumab 40 mg e.o.w. plus DMARDs including MTX, sulfasalazine, leflunomide, intramuscular gold, and hydroxychloroquine, including combinations of DMARDs.

STAR	Treatment (**n**)	ACR 20	ACR 50	ACR 70
	Adalimumab/DMARD (315)	53%*	29%*	15%*
	Placebo/DMARD (315)	35%	11%	3%

*$P < 0.001$ vs placebo.

ReAct (Research in Active Rheumatoid Arthritis trial) – Europe, Australia, Phase IV open-label study [6] Adalimumab 40 mg every other week either as monotherapy or in addition to DMARDs including MTX, sulfasalazine, leflunomide, intramuscular or oral gold, hydroxychloroquine or chloroquine (antimalarials), and azathioprine, either singly or in combination, excluding ciclosporin. 6610 patients were enrolled and followed for 12 weeks in detail, with subsequent voluntary continuation up to 5 years (median follow-up 211 days, maximum 669 days), representing 4210 patient-years of adalimumab exposure.

- 6610 patients enrolled, female 81%; RF-positive 73%; concomitant glucocorticoids 71%.
- Following data are mean(SD): age 54(13) years; previous DMARDs, 3(1.8); DAS28 6.0(1.1); HAQ-DI 1.64(0.68); CRP 26(31); total joint count (TJC) 14(7); swollen joint count (SJC) 10(6).
- Concomitant DMARDs: none, 1731; one DMARD, 4879; MTX, 2794; leflunomide (Lef), 842; antimalarials (AM), 148; sulfasalazine (SSP), 133; other DMARDs, 84.
- Two DMARDs, 769; MTX/Lef, 180; MTX/AM, 269; MTX/SSP, 182.
- Three DMARDs, 106; MTX/SSP/AM, 76.
- At week 12, 7% of enrolled patients withdrew, 4.3% for adverse events and 1.4% for RA activity.

ReAct: week 12

Treatment (*n*)	ACR 20	ACR 50	ACR 70
Adalimumab alone (1731)	60%	32%	15%
Adalimumab + 1 DMARD (4004)	73%	43%	19%

The results were used to assess the odds of achieving RA disease improvement with different combinations of adalimumab and DMARDs versus adalimumab and MTX in combination.

ReAct: week 12 – odds ratios compared with adalimumab and MTX

Adalimumab +	ACR 20	ACR 50	Remission (DAS28 <2.6)
No DMARD	0.52 (0.45–0.60) $P<0.0001$	0.61 (0.53–0.70) $P<0.0001$	0.59 (0.49–0.71) $P<0.0001$
Leflunomide	0.69 (0.58–0.82) $P<0.0001$	0.72 (0.61–0.86) $P=0.0002$	0.75 (0.6–0.93) $P=0.0103$
Sulfasalazine	0.61 (0.41–0.89) $P=0.0112$	0.76 (0.52–1.11) $P=0.1555$	1.51 (0.97–2.36) $P=0.0694$

(continued) ReAct: week 12 – odds ratios compared with adalimumab and MTX

Adalimumab +	ACR 20	ACR 50	Remission (DAS28 <2.6)
Antimalarials	0.86 (0.58–1.26) $P=0.492$	1.14 (0.81–1.63) $P=0.4503$	1.03 (0.65–1.62) $P=0.9107$
Combinations: MTX + Lef	0.67 (0.46–0.96) $P=0.0233$	0.70 (0.50–0.97) $P=0.0307$	0.82 (0.53–1.25) $P=0.3491$

ACR 70 results were similar to those for ACR 20/50.

Values are odds ratios (OR) (95% confidence intervals). All other combinations have OR = 1, with CI including 1, so not significantly different from adalimumab and MTX.

These data support the findings from the PREMIER study that the adalimumab–MTX combination has important disease-suppressing properties compared with adalimumab alone. They also suggest that it may be superior to the combination of adalimumab and leflunomide, with the combination of adalimumab and sulfasalazine having intermediate results.

Serious adverse event (SAE) rates were compared. RA-related events were the most frequent category. SAE rates for adalimumab and single DMARDs were: AM 4.1%; MTX 4.6%; Lef 8.2%; SSP 9.0%.

Serious infection rates were similar to those with adalimumab alone (1.7%): MTX 1.1%; Lef 1.9%; AM 2.0%; SSP 2.3%. Cutaneous and subcutaneous adverse events were reported in 17.3% of patients receiving adalimumab and leflunomide, with 0.8% classified as SAEs. Skin SAEs were not reported with SSP and AM, with 0.1% reported in those receiving adalimumab and MTX.

The SAE rate in patients receiving adalimumab and combinations of MTX and DMARDs was lower than in groups receiving adalimumab and single DMARDs. The experience of tuberculosis screening and infections in this study is summarized in the section on TNF safety.

Conclusion The conclusion of these studies is that adalimumab is efficacious as monotherapy, but the combination of adalimumab and methotrexate has at least additive properties. Adalimumab can be used with most DMARDs and combinations of DMARDs. It significantly reduces progression of radiographic joint damage in patients with rheumatoid arthritis. High levels of remission are achieved in combination with MTX in patients with early RA. Dose increases to adalimumab 40 mg weekly have not been shown to have significant clinical benefit.

Clinical trial data – psoriatic arthritis

ADEPT – USA and Europe, Phase III [7] Randomized 1 : 1 adalimumab 40 mg every other week versus placebo injections. Active PsA defined by SJC ≥3 and TJC ≥3, with concurrent skin psoriasis or a documented history of skin psoriasis. Patients had lack of response or intolerance to at least one non-steroidal anti-inflammatory drug (NSAID). MTX was permitted if taken for at least 3 months, stable for at least 1 month, maximum dose 30 mg/week, and prednisolone no more than 10 mg daily. Tacrolimus, ciclosporin, other DMARDs, or retinoids not permitted within 4 weeks, or any previous treatment with TNF-blockers. Topical therapies for psoriasis were not permitted, except for medicated shampoos or low-potency steroid preparations. Primary efficacy assessments were ACR 20 at week 12 based on a 78/76 joint count, and change in a modified Sharp score of hand and feet radiographs at week 24.

Patients, mean age 49 years, 55.6% male, duration psoriatic arthritis 9.5 ± 8.5 years, duration of psoriasis 17.1 ± 12.3 years. Clinical subtypes: DIP joint arthritis 7.4%; symmetrical polyarticular 67%; asymmetrical arthritis 24.6%; arthritis mutilans 0.3% (one patient); spondylitis 0.3%. 50% were taking MTX.

ADEPT	Treatment (*n*)	ACR 20	ACR 50	ACR 70	HAQ
	Adalimumab 40 mg e.o.w. (151)				
	3 months	58%*	36%*	20%*	−0.4*
	6 months	58%*	39%*	23%*	−0.4*
	Placebo (162)				
	3 months	14%	4%	1%	−0.1
	6 months	14%	6%	1%	−0.1

e.o.w., every other week.

ADEPT	Treatment (*n*)	Change in fatigue Facit-F score	Change in X-ray score
	Adalimumab 40 mg e.o.w. (151) 3 months	7.1*	−0.2*
	Placebo (162) 3 months	0.1	+1.0

e.o.w., every other week.

ADEPT	Treatment (n)	PASI 50	PASI 75	PASI 90	DLQI
	Adalimumab 40 mg e.o.w. (69)				
	3 months	72%*	49%*	30%*	
	6 months	75%*	59%*	42%*	−6.1*
	Placebo (62)				
	3 months	15%	4%	0%	
	6 months	12%	1%	0%	−0.7

PASI, Psoriasis Area and Severity Index (score).
*$P<0.001$ adalimumab vs placebo.
DLQI, Dermatology Quality of Life Index.

There was no apparent effect of concomitant MTX on the clinical responses of either joint or skin outcomes.

Clinical trial data – ankylosing spondylitis

ATLAS – USA, Europe [8] Randomized 2 : 1 adalimumab 40 mg e.o.w. vs placebo injections, over 24 weeks. Patients with AS meeting the modified New York criteria (stable psoriasis, inflammatory bowel disease, reactive arthritis, or uveitis allowed), failed at least one NSAID (inadequate response or toxicity). Criteria for entry, two of three: BASDAI ≥4; total back pain score (visual analogue 10-cm scale) ≥4; duration of early morning stiffness ≥1 hour. Ankylosis of lateral cervical/lumbar spine limited to <10% total population. Stable methotrexate, sulfasalazine, hydroxychloroquine, leflunomide, NSAID, glucocorticoids allowed. Patients on/previously treated with other DMARDs or TNF-blockers excluded. Primary assessments at week 12, patients not achieving ASAS 20 responses at weeks 12, 16, or 20 were offered open-label escape option. Results shown as intention-to-treat, with patients withdrawing from study or with missing values considered as non-responders.

Approx 75% male, mean age approx 42.3 years, mean disease duration approx 10.9 years, BASDAI (mean) approx 6.3, concomitant DMARD approx 20%.

ATLAS	Treatment (n)	ASAS 20/40 responders	Partial remission	Patient global change (0–10 VAS)	Change in BASDAI
	Adalimumab 40 mg e.o.w. (208)	58.2/39.9%*	20.7%*	−39.1%*	−2.6*
	Placebo (107)	20.6/13.1%	3.7%	+6.5	−0.8

e.o.w., every other week; VAS, visual analogue scale. *$P<0.001$ vs placebo.

ATLAS	Treatment (*n*)	Total back pain (0–10 VAS)	ASQoL change	Physician global change (0–10 VAS)	BASDAI 50
	Adalmumab 40 mg e.o.w. (208)	−40.5*	−3.1*	−2.5*	45.2*
	Placebo (107)	−9.5	−1.0	−1.0	15.9

e.o.w., every other week; *$P<0.001$ vs placebo.

Week 24 results were generally similar to those at week 12. Enthesitis score using the Maastricht AS Enthesitis Score (MASES) (range 0–13, baseline value approx 6.4), improved significantly at week 12 in the active therapy group compared with placebo (−2.7 vs −1.3, $P=0.018$) and sustained further improvement at week 24 (−3.2 vs −1.6, $P=0.005$).

References

1 Weinblatt ME, Keystone EC, Furst DE, *et al*. Adalimumab, a fully human anti-tumor necrosis factor α monoclonal antibody, for the treatment of rheumatoid arthritis in patients taking concomitant methotrexate: the ARMADA trial. *Arthritis Rheum* 2003; **48**: 35–45.
2 van de Putte LBA, Rau R, Breedveld FC, *et al*. Efficacy and safety of the fully human anti-tumour necrosis factor α monoclonal antibody adalimumab (D2E7) in DMARD refractory patients with rheumatoid arthritis: a 12 week, phase II study. *Ann Rheum Dis* 2003; **62**: 1168–77.
3 Keystone EC, Kavanaugh AF, Sharp JT, *et al*. Radiographic, clinical, and functional outcomes of treatment with adalimumab (a human anti-tumor necrosis factor monoclonal antibody) in patients with active rheumatoid arthritis receiving concomitant methotrexate therapy: a randomized, placebo-controlled, 52-week trial. *Arthritis Rheum* 2004; **50**: 1400–11.
4 Breedveld FC, Weisman MH, Kavanaugh AF, *et al*. The PREMIER study: a multicenter, randomized, double-blind clinical trial of combination therapy with adalimumab plus methotrexate versus methotrexate alone or adalimumab alone in patients with early, aggressive rheumatoid arthritis who had not had previous methotrexate treatment. *Arthritis Rheum* 2006; **54**: 26–37.
5 Furst DE, Schiff MH, Fleischmann RM, *et al*. Adalimumab, a fully human anti tumor necrosis factor-alpha monoclonal antibody, and concomitant standard antirheumatic therapy for the treatment of rheumatoid arthritis: results of STAR (Safety Trial of Adalimumab in Rheumatoid Arthritis). *J Rheumatol* 2003; **30**: 2563–71.
6 Burmester GR, Mariette X, Montecucco C, *et al*. Adalimumab alone and in combination with disease-modifying antirheumatic drugs for the treatment of rheumatoid arthritis in clinical practice: the Research in Active Rheumatoid Arthritis (ReAct) trial. *Ann Rheum Dis* 2007; **66**: 732–9.

7 Gladman DD, Mease PJ, Ritchlin CT, *et al*. Adalimumab for long-term treatment of psoriatic arthritis: forty-eight week data from the adalimumab effectiveness in psoriatic arthritis trial. *Arthritis Rheum* 2007; **56**: 476–8.
8 van der Heijde D, Kivitz A, Schiff MH, *et al*.; ATLAS Study Group. Efficacy and safety of adalimumab in patients with ankylosing spondylitis: results of a multicenter, randomized, double-blind, placebo-controlled trial. *Arthritis Rheum* 2006; **54**: 2136–46.

Etanercept (Enbrel)

Chemical properties	Recombinant human TNF receptor p75 Fc fusion protein.
	There are two receptors for TNF, a 55-kDa protein, TNFR1 (p55), and a 75-kDa protein TNFR2 (p75), which both bind TNF (TNF-α) and also lymphotoxin (TNF-β)
Manufacture	Produced in Chinese Hamster Ovary (CHO) cells
Stability	Stable for at least 36 months if stored in the dark at 2–8°C
Pharmacokinetics	After a single 25-mg subcutaneous injection, maximum peak serum concentration (C_{max}) was 1.1 ± 0.6 µg/ml, time to C_{max} 69 ± 34 hours. Mean (SD) half-life 102(30) hours. After 6 months of 25 mg twice weekly in the same patients ($n=23$), C_{max} was 2.4 ± 1.0 µg/ml, with a 2–7-fold increase in peak serum concentration. The area under the curve (0–72 hours) rose about 4-fold (range 1–17) with repeated dosing. Age and sex had no effect on pharmacokinetics. The effect of renal or hepatic impairment is unknown
Metabolism	Unclear, but thought to be catabolized in a similar manner to normal human immunoglobulin
Drug interactions	There is no information about interactions with MTX

Clinical trial data – rheumatoid arthritis

The main outcome measures for these studies were the American College of Rheumatology response criteria (ACR 20/50/70), denoting an improvement of at least 20%, 50%, or 70% of RA activity.

Phase IIa study [1] A phase IIa study investigated etanercept given subcutaneously (sc) twice per week at doses of 0.25, 2, or 16 mg per m² body surface area in patients with active RA. Significant dose-dependent improvements in RA in disease activity were noted, beginning with the 2 mg/m² dose (doses of 3.5–4 mg), and definite at 16 mg/m² (doses of 23–30 mg). Dosages of 10 and 25 mg twice weekly were subsequently investigated.

Phase IIb study – USA [2] Patients not responding to at least one and fewer than four DMARDs mean previous number of DMARDs: 3.2. One-month washout of DMARD before starting study drug. Mean age approx 52.5 years, 78% female, disease duration 12 years, mean HAQ 1.7. Assessments at 3 and 6 months.

Dose (*n*)	ACR 20	ACR 50	ACR 70	Mean change in HAQ (%)
10 mg twice/week (76)				
3 months	45%*	13%	8%	−30%§
6 months	51%†	24%†	9%	−34%§
25 mg twice/week (78)				
6 months	59%†	41%†	15%†	−39%§
Placebo (80)				
3 months	23%	8%	4%	−8%
6 months	11%	5%	1%	−2%

*$P=0.003$, †$P<0.001$, ‡$P=0.015$, §$P<0.05$ vs placebo group.

Phase III – USA [3] Randomized 2 : 1 to etanercept and MTX versus placebo and MTX, in MTX non-responders. Age approx 50 years, 845 female, disease duration 13 years, 86% RF positive, mean previous DMARDs 2.7. Previously received MTX for at least 6 months, stable dose 12.5–25 mg weekly for at least 4 weeks (96% of patients taking >15 mg).

Dose (*n*)	ACR 20	ACR 50	ACR 70	Change in HAQ
25 mg twice/week (59)				
12 weeks	66%*	42%†	15%†	
24 weeks	71%†	39%†	15%†	−0.7
Placebo (30)				
12 weeks	33%	0%	0%	
24 weeks	27%	3%	0%	−0.4

*$P=0.03$, †$P<0.001$, ‡$P=0.003$ vs placebo group.

Early Rheumatoid Arthritis (ERA) Study – USA, Canada, Phase III [4] Patients with early RA of less than 3 years' duration, no previous MTX. Mean age approx 50 years, 75% female, disease duration 11.7 months. Erosions in 87%, RF-positive 88%. Patients received etanercept 10 or 25 mg, or placebo injections twice per week, plus MTX starting at 7.5 mg per week, increasing to 20 mg by week 8 (average dose 19 mg week 20).

Dose (n)	ACR 20	ACR 50	ACR 70	X-ray change (total Sharp score/ erosion score)
10 mg twice/week (208)				
3 months	58%	29%	6%	Similar to MTX
6 months	58%	33%	13%	Similar to MTX
12 months	63%	32%	15%	Similar to MTX
25 mg twice/week (207)				
3 months	62%	29%	13%*	ND
6 months	65%	40%	21%	0.57/0.30†
12 months	72%	49%	25%	1.00/0.47‡
MTX (217)				
3 months	56%	24%	7%	ND
6 months	58%	32%	14%	1.06/0.68
12 months	65%	43%	22%	1.59/1.03

*P < 0.05, †P < 0.01, ‡P < 0.02 vs MTX group. ND, not determined.

TEMPO – USA, Canada, Europe, Australia [5] Failed at least one DMARD other than MTX. If previous MTX, then none for at least 6 months and no previous clinically important toxicity or lack of response. Mean age 53 years, female 77%, mean disease duration 6.6 (SD 5) years. Mean dose MTX after week 8, 17.2 mg/week MTX monotherapy, 16.9 mg/week combination group. Clinical outcomes, remission defined by Disease Activity Score less than 1.6, and radiographic outcomes, both at week 52.

TEMPO	Treatment (n)	ACR 50	DAS remission	Change in vdH/ Sharp score mean	Change in HAQ
	MTX alone (228)	43%	13%	2.8	−0.6
	Etanercept alone, 25 mg twice/week (223)	48%	16%	0.52‡	−0.7
	MTX + etanercept (231)	69%*	35%*	−0.54†	−1.0*

*P < 0.0001 vs MTX alone and etanercept alone.
†P < 0.0001 vs MTX alone, P < 0.0006 vs etanercept alone.
‡P < 0.0077 vs MTX alone.
vdH, van der Heijde

Etanercept 50 mg once-weekly dosing Reconsideration of the pharmacokinetics of etanercept showed that the half-life was compatible with once weekly dosing of 50 mg. A randomized placebo-controlled study compared 50 mg once weekly dosing to the usual 25 mg twice per week [6]. 214 patients received 50 mg etanercept once weekly, 153 received 25 mg etanercept twice weekly, and 53 received placebo for 8 weeks followed by 25 mg etanercept twice weekly for 8 weeks. Approximately 50% of patients in each group were taking MTX at a mean dose of 14–15 mg per week. Efficacy and safety were assessed at weeks 8 and 16.

Dose (*n*)	ACR 20	ACR 50	ACR 70	% improvement HAQ	CRP
25 mg twice/week (153)					
8 weeks	49%*	18%†	5%†	29.7	17.0
16 weeks	63%	33%	8%	37.3	27.3
50 mg once/week (214)					
8 weeks	50%*	18%†	2%	33.0	21.9
16 weeks	55%	29%	8%	35.4	14.5
Placebo (53), 8 weeks	19%	6%	2%	−7.7	−41.0

*$P < 0.001$, †$P = 0.03$ vs placebo.

Adverse effects were similar, including injection site reactions occurring in 19% of patients in both the 25-mg twice weekly and 50-mg once weekly groups by week 16 (6% in placebo group at week 8). Pharmacokinetics were similar with mean area under the curve (AUC) of 297 g.hours/litre in the 50-mg group and 317 mg.hours/litre in the 25-mg twice-weekly group.

Etanercept in combination with anakinra [7] Etanercept 25 mg twice weekly plus daily anakinra or placebo injections for 6 months. Patients with active RA despite MTX. Patients were randomized 1:1:1 to 25 mg etanercept twice weekly and placebo anakinra, 25 mg etanercept once weekly plus anakinra 100 mg daily, etanercept 25 mg twice weekly plus anakinra 100 mg daily. Patient approximate mean values: 72% female, age 54 years, disease duration 10 years, MTX 16 mg/week. HAQ 1.5, 49% on glucocorticosteroids, SJC 21, TJC 33, ESR 48.

Dose (*n*)	ACR 20	ACR 50	ACR 70	Serious infections	Injection site reactions
Anakinra + etanercept					
25 mg twice/week (81), 6 months	62%	31%	14%	7%	70%
Anakinra + etanercept					
25 mg once/week (80), 6 months	51%	39%	24%	4%	68%
Placebo + etanercept					
25 mg twice/week (80), 6 months	68%	41%	21%	0%	40%

$P = 0.037$ vs etanercept once/week + anakinra.

Phase IV etanercept and sulfasalazine – Europe [8] Patients with active RA despite sulfasalazine therapy (2–3 g daily) [6]. Randomized study of sulfasalazine and placebo injections versus sulfasalazine and etanercept versus etanercept alone. 24-week study.

Sulfasalazine and Etanercept Study

Treatment (n)	ACR 20	ACR 50	ACR 70	Change in HAQ
Sulfasalazine + placebo injection (50)	28%	13%	2%	−0.1
Etanercept alone 25 mg twice/week (103)	74%*	16%	21%	−0.6
Sulfasalazine + etanercept (101)	74%*	35%	25%	−0.6

*$P<0.05$ vs sulfasalazine.

Phase IV: etanercept in active very early rheumatoid arthritis – COMET Study [9] Primary outcome measure was remission assessed by DAS28 score <2.6 after 52 weeks of etanercept and MTX versus MTX alone. Patients with active RA of less than 2 years' duration, no previous MTX, DAS28 score >3.2, and ESR ≥28 mm/hour or CRP ≥20 mg/litre. Mean age 51 years, median disease duration 7 months, mean DAS28 6.1, 22% had previous DMARDs.

COMET Study	Treatment (n)	DAS 28 remission	Low DAS (2.7–3.2)	ACR 50	ACR 70
	MTX alone (268)	28%	41%	49%	28%
	MTX + etanercept (274)	50%*	64%*	71%*	48%*

*$P<0.001$ vs MTX alone.

Etanercept 100 mg per week versus 50 mg per week [10] Seventy-seven patients with RA were randomized (2:1) to receive either 50 mg (51 patients) or 25 mg (26 patients) of etanercept twice a week for 24 weeks. No difference was detected between the two groups in the primary outcome measure, the ACR-N AUC at 24 weeks. Likewise, no difference in ACR 20, 50, and 70, or European League Against Rheumatism (EULAR) response criteria were seen. There were no significant differences between the two groups in non-infectious adverse events. However, there was a significant increase in upper respiratory tract infections in patients receiving 100 mg etanercept versus those receiving 50 mg (26% vs 4%, $P=0.027$).

The conclusion of these studies is that etanercept is efficacious as monotherapy, but the combination of etanercept and MTX has at least additive properties. Etanercept significantly reduces progression of radiographic joint damage in patients with RA. High levels of remission are achieved in combination with MTX in patients with mild RA who have received no or little previous MTX. Etanercept can be used as 50 mg once per week with similar results to 25 mg twice per week, although the incidence of injection site reactions is similar. Etanercept 100 mg per week is no better than 50 mg per week and has a higher risk of upper respiratory tract infections. Etanercept is not recommended in combination with either anakinra or abatacept (details in Abatacept section), as no added efficacy is achieved and increased rates of infectious adverse events are seen.

Clinical trial data – psoriatic arthritis

Phase II USA randomized 1:1 etanercept 25 mg twice per week versus placebo injections [11] Patients with active PsA defined by SJC ≥3 and TJC ≥3, who had failed NSAID therapy and were candidates for DMARD therapy. Current significant skin psoriasis not mandatory. MTX 47% of patients, stable for at least 4 weeks, maximum dose 25 mg/week. Median age 45 years, approx 51% male, assessment at 12 weeks.

Etanercept dose (n)	ACR 20	ACR 50	ACR 70	Change in HAQ	PsARC
25 mg twice/week (30), 12 weeks	73%*	50% †	13% ‡	−1.2*	87%*
Placebo (30), 12 weeks	13%	3%	0%	−0.1	23%

*$P < 0.0001$, †$P = 0.001$, ‡$P = 0.0403$ vs placebo.
PsARC, Psoriatic Arthritis Response Criteria.

Etanercept dose (n)	Change in TJC (0–78)	Change in SJC (0–76)	Change in CRP (mg/l)	PASI 50	PASI 75
25 mg twice/week (30), 12 weeks	−16.5*	−11.0*	−10*	36%	26%†
Placebo (30), 12 weeks	+3.5	−3.7	+2	18%	0%

*$P < 0.0002$, †$P = 0.0154$.
PASI, Psoriasis Area and Severity Index.

Phase III – USA, Canada [12] Randomized 1:1 etanercept 25 mg twice per week versus placebo injections. Patients active PsA defined by SJC =3 and TJC =3, who had failed NSAID therapy, in one or more of the following clinical subtypes: distal interphalangeal (DIPI) joint arthritis ($n = 104$), polyarticular with psoriasis, absent RF ($n = 173$), arthritis mutilans ($n = 3$), asymmetrical arthritis ($n=81$), or AS like ($n=7$). In addition, skin psoriasis with a target lesion at least 2 cm in diameter should be present. MTX stable for at least 2 months, maximum dose 25 mg/week was permitted; average dose in placebo group 15.4 mg per week, etanercept group 16.3 mg per week. Mean age 47.5 years, 51% male, assessment at 6 months.

Etanercept dose (n)	ACR 20	ACR 50	ACR 70	Change in HAQ	PsARC
25 mg twice/week (101)					
3 months	59%*	40%*	9%*		72%*
6 months	50%*	37%*	9%*	−0.8*	70%*
Placebo (104)					
3 months	15%	5%	0%		31%
6 months	13%	4%	1%	−0.1	23%

*$P<0.0001$ vs placebo.

Etanercept dose (n)	Change in TJC (0–78)	Change in SJC (0–76)	Change in pain (0–5)	Global change in physician (0–5)	Change in CRP (mg/l)
25 mg twice/week (101), 6 months	−13*	−8*	−2*	−2*	−14*
Placebo (104), 6 months	−4	−3	0	0	0

*$P<0.0001$ vs placebo.

Etanercept dose (n)	PASI 50	PASI 75
25 mg twice/week (66), 6 months	47%*	23%*
Placebo (62), 6 months	18%	3%

PASI, Psoriasis Area and Severity Index (score).

*$P<0.001$ vs placebo.

Etanercept dose (n)	Change in total X-ray score
25 mg twice/week (101), 12 months	−0.3*
Placebo (104), 12 months	+1.00

*$P<0.0001$ vs placebo.

There was no apparent effect of concomitant MTX on the clinical responses for either joint or skin outcomes.

Clinical trial data – ankylosing spondylitis

Etanercept has been studied in three placebo-controlled trials in AS, using 25-mg injections twice weekly versus placebo injections. Two initial placebo-controlled studies with small numbers of patients were followed by a larger study.

Gorman et al. [13] Patients with AS meeting the modified New York criteria and inflammatory back pain, active as defined by duration of early morning stiffness more than 45 min, plus VAS ≥40 for physician global assessment (0–100) and patient global assessment at least moderate on a 1–5 scale; DMARDs, NSAIDs, and glucocorticoids continued at a stable dose. 16-week assessments.

Gorman et al. [13]

Treatment (n)	Change in early morning stiffness	Night pain (VAS)	Change in BASDAI	Change in BASFI	Modified Newcastle Enthesitis Index
Etanercept 25 mg twice/week (20)	90 min, reduced to 25 min*	−50*	−1.0*	−2.3*	−4.5*
Placebo (20)	60 min, no change	−8.5	−0	−0.1	−1.5

*$P<0.01$ vs placebo.

Patients were then enrolled in an open-label extension study for 10 months, with similar improvements in those receiving placebo and maintenance of initial responses in the active treatment group.

Brandt et al. [14] Investigator-initiated study, Germany. Glucocorticoids and DMARDs stopped 4 weeks before treatment. Thirty patients (active/placebo), average age 40/32 years, 70%/75% male, 86%/94% HLA-B27-positive disease, duration 14.9/11.4 years, BASDAI 6.5/6.6. Placebo-controlled for 6 weeks, then active therapy until week 12 in active group and week 18 in placebo group, so each group received etanercept for 12 weeks. After drug cessation patients were followed for 12 weeks. Assessment at 6 weeks.

Brandt et al. [14]

Treatment (n)	BASDAI 50	ASAS 20/50	Change in BASDAI	Change in BASFI	Change in BASMI
Etanercept 25 mg twice/week (14)	57%*	78.6%/42.9%†	−3.0‡	−1.9§	−1.5#
Placebo (16)	1%	25%/12.5%	−0.8	−0.2	−0.3

*$P<0.004$, †$P<0.01$, ‡$P=0.003$, §$P=0.008$, #$P=0.01$ vs placebo.

Significantly more patients receiving etanercept reduced their NSAID dose by 50% compared with those receiving placebo. Non-significant reductions in peripheral arthritis or enthesitis were noted in the small number of patients with these disease manifestations. Twenty-four patients from the total group of 30 who achieved at least a BASDAI 20 response to etanercept were observed after cessation of treatment. Of these, 18 (75%) experienced a relapse of symptoms (defined as an increase of 2 or more in their BASDAI score) within the 6-week observation period. The remainder of the patients all relapsed at a later time.

Phase III – USA, Canada, and Europe. Davis *et al*. [15] Patients aged between 18 and 70 years, AS meeting the modified New York criteria, active as defined by presence of VAS score ≥30 for average and duration of early morning stiffness, plus VAS ≥30 for two of three following parameters: patient global assessment; average of VAS scores for nocturnal and total back pain; average of 10 questions on the Bath Ankylosing Spondylitis Functional Index (BASFI). Continued to receive DMARDs, NSAIDs, and glucocorticoids at a stable dose. Primary outcome measure was the ASAS 20 response at 6 months. The ASAS 20 response measure is the ASsessment of Ankylosing Spondylitis criteria of ≥20% improvement in at least three of the following criteria: patient global score; back pain; BASFI, with no worsening of the other domains. ASAS 50 and 70 responses are defined in a similar way.

Average age 42 years, disease duration 10.3 years, 76% male, 84% HLA-B27, 91% taking NSAIDs, 31% taking DMARDs, 4.5% Crohn's disease, 9.5% psoriasis, 30% uveitis, BASDAI score: active therapy group, 59.6; placebo group, 58.1.

Phase III	Treatment (*n*)	ASAS 20	ASAS 50	ASAS 70	Partial remission
	Etanercept 25 mg twice/week (138)				
	2 weeks	46%*	24%*	12%†	
	3 months	59%*	45%*	29%†	17%
	6 months	57%*	42%*	28%†	
	Placebo (139)				
	2 weeks	22%	7%	2%	
	3 months	28%	13%	7%	4%
	6 months	22%	10%	5%	

*$P<0.0001$, †$P=0.002$ vs placebo.

Phase III

Treatment (*n*)	Change in BASFI	Pt global change (0–10 VAS)	Change in BASDAI	Total back pain (0–10 VAS)
Etanercept 25mg (65) twice/week (138)	−15.7*	−20*	−23.6*	−20.7*
Placebo (139)	−4.6	0	−4.5	−2.4

* $P < 0.0001$ vs placebo.

Concomitant DMARDs did not influence the clinical response.

More recently it has been shown that etanercept 50 mg subcutaneously once per week has equal efficacy in AS to the previously studied dose of 25 mg twice weekly [16].

References

1 Moreland LW, Baumgartner SW, Schiff MH, *et al*. Treatment of rheumatoid arthritis with a recombinant human tumor necrosis factor receptor (p75)-Fc fusion protein. *N Engl J Med* 1997; **337**: 141–7.

2 Moreland LW, Schiff MH, Baumgartner SW, *et al*. Etanercept therapy in rheumatoid arthritis: a randomized, controlled trial. *Ann Intern Med* 1999; **130**: 478–86.

3 Weinblatt ME, Kremer JM, Bankhurst AD, *et al*. A trial of etanercept, a recombinant tumor necrosis factor receptor:Fc fusion protein in patients with rheumatoid arthritis receiving methotrexate. *N Engl J Med* 1999; **340**: 253–9.

4 Bathon JM, Martin RW, Fleischmann RM, *et al*. A comparison of etanercept and methotrexate in patients with early rheumatoid arthritis. *N Engl J Med* 2000; **343**: 1586–93.

5 Klareskog L, van der Heijde D, de Jager JP, *et al*. Therapeutic effect of the combination of etanercept and methotrexate compared with each treatment alone in patients with rheumatoid arthritis: double-blind randomised controlled trial. *Lancet* 2004; **363**: 675–81.

6 Keystone E, Schiff M, Kremer J, *et al*. Once-weekly administration of 50 mg etanercept in patients with active rheumatoid arthritis: results of a multicenter, randomized, double-blind, placebo-controlled trial. *Arthritis Rheum* 2004; **50**: 353–63.

7 Genovese MC, Cohen S, Moreland L, *et al*. Combination therapy with etanercept and anakinra in the treatment of patients with rheumatoid arthritis who have been treated unsuccessfully with methotrexate. *Arthritis Rheum* 2004; **50**: 1412–19.

8 Combe B, Codreanu C, Fiocco U, *et al*., for the Etanercept European Investigators Network. Etanercept and sulfasalazine, alone and combined, in patients with active rheumatoid arthritis despite receiving sulfasalazine: a double-blind comparison. *Ann Rheum Dis* 2006; **65**: 1357–62.

9 Emery P, Breedveld, F, Hall S, *et al*. Remission rates in subjects with active early rheumatoid arthritis – 1 year results of the COMET trial: COmbination of Methotrexate and ETanercept in active early rheumatoid arthritis. Late breaking abstract ACR/AHRP Scientific Meeting November 2007. No. L17.

10 Johnsen AK, Schiff MH, Mease PJ, *et al*. Comparison of 2 doses of etanercept (50 vs 100 mg) in active rheumatoid arthritis: a randomized double blind study. *J Rheumatol* 2006; **33**: 659–64.

11 Mease PJ, Goffe BS, Metz J, VanderStoep A, Finck B, and Burge DJ. Etanercept in the treatment of psoriatic arthritis and psoriasis: a randomised trial. *Lancet* 2000; **356**: 385–90.

12 Mease PJ, Kivitz AJ, Burch FX, *et al*. Etanercept treatment of psoriatic arthritis: safety, efficacy, and effect on disease progression. *Arthritis Rheum* 2004; **50**: 2264–72.

13 Gorman JD, Sack KE, and Davis JC. Treatment of ankylosing spondylitis by inhibition of tumor necrosis factor alpha. *N Engl J Med* 2002; **346**: 1349–56.

14 Brandt J, Khariouzov A, Listing J, *et al*. Six-month results of a double-blind, placebo-controlled trial of etanercept treatment in patients with active ankylosing spondylitis. *Arthritis Rheum* 2003; **48**: 1667–75.

15 Davis JC, van der Heijde D, Braun J, *et al*. Recombinant human tumor necrosis factor receptor (etanercept) for treating ankylosing spondylitis: a randomized, controlled trial. *Arthritis Rheum* 2003; **48**: 3230–6.

16 van der Heijde D, Da Silva JC, Dougados M, *et al*; Etanercept Study 314 Investigators. Etanercept 50 mg once weekly is as effective as 25 mg twice weekly in patients with ankylosing spondylitis. *Ann Rheum Dis* 2006; **65**: 1572–7.

Infliximab (Remicade)

Administration	Intravenous infusion in normal saline (sodium chloride 0.9%) over 2 hours
Chemical properties	Recombinant human–murine chimaeric IgG1 monoclonal antibody
Manufacture	Produced in cell line by continuous perfusion
Stability	Stable for at least 36 months if stored in the dark at 2–8°C
Pharmacokinetics	Single dose of 3–10 mg/kg in RA and 5 mg/kg in Crohn's disease, indicating a median terminal half-life of 8–9.5 days. Single 3–20 mg/kg intravenous dosage showed linear dose–blood level relationship, indicating mainly intravascular compartment distribution. Eight weeks after a dose given during regular therapy, stable blood levels of approximately 0.5–6 µg/ml were seen, with no systemic accumulation of drug. A trough level >1 µg/ml is associated with good clinical responses in RA. The development of anti-infliximab antibodies substantially increased clearance. However, antibodies do not explain most of the variability in rates of clearance seen in many patients, which is currently poorly explained
Metabolism	Unclear but thought to be catabolized in a similar manner to normal human immunoglobulin
Drug interactions	MTX and other immunosuppressant medications probably decrease the formation of antibodies against infliximab and increase plasma concentrations of infliximab

Clinical trial data – rheumatoid arthritis

Phase II/III studies The main outcome measures for these studies were the American College of Rheumatology response criteria (ACR 20/50/70), denoting an improvement of at least 20%, 50%, or 70% of RA activity. These studies were performed in the USA and Europe, and are summarized below.

Elliott et al. [1,2] An initial open-label study of infliximab [1] was tested in a randomized double-blind study of a single infusion of either 1 or 10 mg/kg versus placebo in 73 patients with active RA who had failed many previous DMARDs.

The primary outcome measure was the Paulus 20% response criteria, a composite response measure of six clinical or laboratory measures. Two of 24 placebo-treated patients responded, compared with 11 of 24 patients receiving 1 mg/kg and 19 of 24 receiving 10 mg/kg, a highly significant response $P<0.0001$. More than half of the high-dose group achieved a Paulus 50% response ($P=0.0005$).

ATTRACT – USA, Europe [3,4] Patients not responding to MTX, median dose in active therapy group 15 mg, placebo group 15 mg per week. Median age 54 years, 72% female, median disease duration 8.4 years. Subjects randomized to five different treatment groups: infliximab 3 or 10 mg/kg or placebo, at weeks 0, 2, and 6, and then either every 4 or 8 weeks for 102 weeks. Assessments at 30, 54, and 102 weeks.

ATTRACT week 54

Dose (*n*)	ACR 20	ACR 50	ACR 70	Change in HAQ-DI	X-ray change* (mean/median)
3 mg/kg					
8 weekly (86)	42%‡	21%†	11%†	−0.4‡	1.3‡/0.5
4 weekly (86)	48%‡	34%‡	18%‡	−0.5‡	1.6‡/0.1
10 mg/kg					
8 weekly (87)	59%‡	40%‡	26%‡	−0.5‡	0.2‡/0.5
4 weekly (81)	59%‡	38%‡	19%	−0.4‡	−0.7‡/−0.5
Placebo (88)	17%	9%	2%	−0.2	7.0/4.0

*vdH/Sharp score.
†$P<0.05$, ‡$P<0.001$ vs placebo.

ASPIRE – Europe, USA, Australia, Canada, Phase III [5] MTX-naive patients with RA of <3 years' duration (median 0.6 years). All patients received MTX, increased by week 8 to 20 mg per week, and either infliximab 3 or 6 mg/kg, or placebo, at weeks 0, 2, and 6, then every 8 weeks. Approximately 70% of patients achieved the target dose of MTX of 20 mg/week, mean dose at week 54, 15 mg/week. Assessment at week 54. Mean age 50 years, 70% female [3].
ASPIRE Study: week 54

Dose (n)	ACR 20	ACR 50	ACR 70	Median change in HAQ-DI	X-ray change* (mean/median)
3 mg/kg (351)	62%†	46%§	33%‡	−0.80†	0.42§/0.00
6 mg/kg (355)	66%§	50%§	37%§	−0.88§	0.51§/0.00
Placebo (274)	46%	32%	21%	−0.68	3.7/0.43

*vdH/Sharp score.

†$P < 0.05$, ‡$P < 0.01$, §$P < 0.001$ vs placebo.

ASPIRE Study

	DAS28 week 0	DAS28 week 54	DAS28 remission week 54
Placebo + MTX	6.7	4.6	15%
Infliximab 3 mg/kg + MTX	6.6	4.0†	21%
Infliximab 6 mg/kg + MTX	6.8	3.7*	31%*

*$P < 0.001$, †$P = 0.001$ vs placebo + MTX.

START – Safety Trial for Rheumatoid Arthritis with Remicade (infliximab) Therapy Trial [6] Postmarketing randomized controlled double-blind dose-related safety and dose escalation study. Patients not responding to MTX. Patients randomized, stratified by steroid dose and study centre site, into three groups: group 1, placebo for 22 weeks then 3 mg/kg; group 2, 3 mg/kg until week 22, when dose escalation could occur; group 3, 10 mg/kg.

In group 2, patients not achieving a 20% improvement of baseline SJC and TJC at week 22 (primary non-responders), or who responded at week 22 but later had a disease activity flare, defined as an increase of 50% of week 22 TJC and SJC (secondary non-responders), were allocated progressive dose increases of 1.5 mg/kg. The increases were made in a blinded manner; patients and investigators were not aware of who had received increases in therapy. If disease activity did not respond to the initial increase, further increases of 1.5 mg/kg were made at weeks 30, 38, and 46 for primary non-responders. Secondary non-responders had their first dose increase at week 30. Infliximab and anti-infliximab antibody levels were measured throughout the study. All patients were on stable concomitant MTX, but were also allowed to continue chloroquine, hydroxychloroquine, azathioprine, sulfasalazine, leflunomide, ciclosporin (no more than 5 mg/kg), oral or intramuscular gold, penicillamine, oral corticosteroids, or NSAIDs. Latent tuberculosis (TB) was assessed by purified protein derivative (PPD) skin testing in the USA and according to local guidelines in other countries; isoniazid was given if latent TB suspected.

Median age 52 years, 80% female, disease duration (median) 7.5 years, average MTX dose (all groups) 15 mg per week. Approximately 25% and 4.7% of patients in all groups took either one or two DMARDs, respectively, in addition to MTX. Some 59% of patients took corticosteroids. Patients with conditions that might predispose them to infections such as diabetes (5.4%), chronic respiratory infection/bronchiectasis (0.4%), chronic renal failure (0.2%), osteomyelitis and chronic renal infection (both 0.1%), were distributed evenly between the groups, making up 8.0%, 8.1%, and 5.5% of the patients in groups 1, 2, and 3, respectively.

The primary endpoint was the occurrence of serious infection in the three treatment groups at week 22. Last measurements were made at week 54.

START Study: week 22 data

	Dose (*n*)	Serious infection	Relative risk vs group 1	*P*
Group 1	Placebo (363)	6 (1.7%)		
Group 2	3 mg/kg (360)	6 (1.7%)	1.0 (95% CI 0.3–3.1)	0.995
Group 3	10 mg/kg (361)	18 (5.0%)	3.1 (95% CI 1.2–7.9)	0.013

START Study: week 22 data

	Dose (*n*)	ACR 20	ACR 50	ACR 70	DAS28 (good/mod)	DAS28 remission
Group 1	Placebo (363)	26%	9.7%	4.7%	44%	14%
Group 2	3 mg/kg (360)	58%*	32.1%*	14.0%*	75%*	31%*
Group 3	10 mg/kg (361)	61%*	35.4%*	16.1%*	79%*	32%*

*$P < 0.001$ vs group 1 (MTX plus placebo).

START dose escalation: responders (20% reduction of SJC and TJC)

	Primary non-responders (53)		Secondary non-responders (47)	
One increase	4.5 mg/kg (23)	86.4%	4.5 mg/kg (36)	83.3%
Two increases	6.0 mg/kg (13)	81.0%	6.0 mg/kg (8)	75 0%
Three increases	7.5 mg/kg (10)	90.0%	7.5 mg/kg (3)	100.0%
Four increases	9.0 mg/kg (7)	0.0%	Not possible	NA

NA, not available.

In this study, patients not achieving an ACR 20 response or having a later disease flare were eligible for increases in therapy. Approximately two-thirds of patients did not require dose escalation from 3 mg/kg over the 54 weeks of the study. Primary and secondary non-responder groups both responded well to dose increases. This study confirmed previous findings that a trough level of infliximab >1 µg/ml is necessary for optimal responses [3]. Patients who required dose escalation had a non-significant increased incidence of anti-infliximab antibodies compared with patients with stable dose requirements (28.6% vs 19.5%). However, anti-infliximab antibodies were not detected in the majority of patients who required dose increases, despite a more rapid clearance of infliximab (lower trough levels) in these patients.

The seven patients who were primary non-responders and showed no improvement at any time after four dose increases to 9 mg/kg had good week 22 trough infliximab levels (>1 µg/ml), and only one was positive for anti-infliximab antibodies. This group had disease of long duration (mean 12.1 years) with low baseline median CRP levels of 7 mg/l, compared with the median for all group 2 patients of 24 mg/l; the paper suggested they may have had a more non-inflammatory disease process.

There was no significant worsening of adverse events in patients receiving dose increases compared with those who did not. Six patients (5.5%) stopped therapy prematurely because of adverse events, versus seven (3.2%) who did not receive dose escalation.

Overview

The conclusion of these studies is that infliximab is efficacious in combination with MTX. Infliximab is licensed with MTX for the treatment of RA. It significantly reduces progression of radiological joint damage in patients with RA. High levels of remission are achieved in patients with early RA. In both primary or secondary non-responders with established disease, modest (1.5 mg/kg) dose increases at a regular dosing interval improves outcome. Trough serum levels greater than 1 µg/ml predict response, but the reasons why some patients have more rapid clearance of infliximab is unclear.

Clinical trial data – psoriatic arthritis

IMPACT Study – USA, Canada, Europe [7,8] Phase II randomized 1:1 infliximab 5 mg/kg at weeks 0, 2, 6, and 14 versus placebo infusions.

Patients active PsA defined by SJC ≥5 and TJC ≥5, plus early morning stiffness >45 min, or ESR ≥28 mm/hour or CRP ≥15 mg/l. Active skin psoriasis not necessary. Patients should have failed at least one DMARD (inefficacy or tolerability). Glucocorticoids (no more that 10 mg daily), NSAIDs, and all DMARDs with the exception of ciclosporin A and cyclophosphamide permitted at stable doses, 71% of patients. Female 42.3%, age (median) 45.4 years, PsA disease duration 11.3 years, psoriasis disease duration 18.2 years, dactylitis 50%, enthesitis 25%, PASI >2.5, 37.6%. MTX, placebo group 34/52, mean dose 16.2 mg/week; infliximab group 24/52, mean dose 15.9 mg/week.

Primary endpoint assessments at week 16.

IMPACT Study

Treatment (n)	ACR 20	ACR 50	ACR 70	Change in HAQ	PsARC
Infliximab 5 mg/kg (52)	65.4%*	46.2%*	28.8%*	−0.6*	75%*
Placebo (52)	9.6%	0%	0%	0	11%

*$P<0.001$ vs placebo.

IMPACT Study

Treatment (n)	Change in TJC (0–78)	Change in SJC (0–76)	Change in pain (0–5)	Global change in physician (0–100)	Change in CRP (mg/l)
Infliximab 5 mg/kg (52)	−17*	−12*	−35*	−35*	−10*
Placebo (52)	+2	−1	+1	0	−1

*$P<0.001$ vs placebo.

IMPACT Study

Treatment (n)	PASI 50	PASI 75
Infliximab 5 mg/kg (22)	100%*	68%*
Placebo (17)	0%	0%

*$P<0.001$ vs placebo.

Enthesitis score improved by 85% in patients receiving infliximab versus 29% in those receiving placebo ($P<0.001$). Enthesitis, reported by 25% of patients at enrolment, fell to 14% in the active therapy group, but increased to 31% in those receiving placebo ($P=0.021$).

IMPACT 2 Study – USA, Canada, Europe [9] Phase III randomized 1 : 1 infliximab 5mg/kg at weeks 0, 2, 6 then eight weekly week 22 vs placebo infusions [9,10]. All patients received infliximab after week 24 with poor responders receiving 10mg/kg after week 38.

Patients active PsA defined by SJC≥3 and TJC≥3, plus early morning stiffness >45 minutes in one or more of the following clinical subtypes: DIP joint arthritis 25%, polyarticular (50%), arthritis mutilans (1.5%), asymmetric arthritis (20%), or spondylitis and arthritis (4%). Active skin psoriasis necessary, with at least one area >2 cm diameter. Patients should have failed at least one NSAID (inefficacy or tolerability). Glucocorticoids (no more than 10 mg daily), NSAIDs and all DMARDs excluded with the exception of methotrexate (46%). Female 39%, age (mean) 47 years, PsA disease duration (mean) 8 years, subject with less than or equal to 3% body Surface Area Psoriasis 85%, Swollen Joint Count (0–66) 14, Tender Joint Count (0–68) 25.

IMPACT 2

Treatment (n)		ACR 20	ACR 50	ACR 70	HAQ (% achieving MCID)†	PsARC
Infliximab 5 mg/kg	Week 14 (100)	58%*	36%*	15%*	(59%)*	77%*
	Week 24 (83)	54%*	41%*	27%*	(52%)*	70%*
Placebo	Week 14 (100)	11%	3%	1%	(19%)	27%
	Week 24 (87)	16%	4%	2%	(20%)	32%

*$P<0.001$ active therapy compared to placebo.
†MCID – minimum clinically important difference.

IMPACT 2

Treatment (n)		PASI 50	PASI 75
Infliximab 5 mg/kg	Week 14 (83)	82%*	64%*
	Week 24 (83)	75%*	60%*
Placebo	Week 14 (87)	9%	2%
	Week 24 (87)	8%	1%

*$P<0.001$ active therapy compared to placebo.

IMPACT 2

Treatment (n)		Change in X-ray score†	Radiographic progression‡
Infliximab 5 mg/kg (100)	Week 24	−0.70 ± 2.53*	12%
	Week 54	−0.94 ± 3.4*	8%
Placebo (100)	Week 24	+0.82 ± 2.62	3%
	Week 54	+0.53 ± 2.60	1%

*$P<0.001$ active therapy compared to placebo.
†Mean ± SD Sharp/van der Heijde score modified for PsA.
‡Change greater than smallest detectable change.

Dactylitis was reported by 39% of patients at baseline and fell to 19% and 15% at weeks 14 and 24, respectively, in the infliximab group, significantly better than the stable occurrence of 32% and 33% in the placebo group ($P<0.05$).

Enthesitis, reported by approximately 39% of patients at enrolment, at week 14 fell to 22.2% in the active therapy group, compared with 33.7% in those receiving placebo ($P=0.016$), and at week 24 was 20.4% in infliximab group versus 37.2% in for placebo ($P=0.002$).

Clinical trial data – ankylosing spondylitis

PO1522 – Germany [10] Phase IIb, investigator-initiated, placebo-controlled trial. Weeks 0–12 randomized 1:1 to either placebo ($n=35$) or infliximab 5 mg/kg ($n=35$) on weeks 0, 2, 6, and 12. Then an open-label comparative study with infliximab 5 mg/kg every 6 weeks for all patients to week 24. Long-term extension study from weeks 54–102 included 53 patients.

Marked improvement seen in all markers of signs and symptoms of AS in active therapy group compared with placebo. Improvements noted after 2 weeks, and maintained to week 54, and then in the long-term extension study to 102 weeks.

PO1522 week 12

Treatment (n)	BASDAI 50	Partial remission	Patient global change (0–10 VAS)	Change in BASDAI
Infliximab 5 mg/kg (35)	53%*	68%*	18%*	–3.4%*
Placebo (35)	9%	25%	0%	–0.8%

*$P<0.001$ vs placebo.

ASSERT – USA, Canada, Europe [11] Phase III randomized 8:3 infliximab 5 mg/kg IV weeks 0, 2, 6, 12, and 18 versus placebo injections; primary endpoint at 24 weeks [12].

Patients with AS meeting the modified New York criteria (stable inflammatory bowel disease, psoriasis, or uveitis allowed). Criteria for entry, two of three: BASDAI ≥4; total back pain score (VAS 10-cm scale) >4; duration of early morning stiffness >1 hour. Ankylosis of lateral thoracolumbar spine excluded on radiography. Stable NSAIDs only, all DMARDs and systemic glucocorticoids stopped prior to study.

Male approx 80.6%, age (median) 40 years, disease duration (median) 8.8 years, 87% HLA-B27 positive, proportion with history of uveitis (median) approx 34.5%, inflammatory bowel disease approx 7.3%, and psoriasis approx 7.4%, BASDAI (median) approx 6.5.

ASSERT week 24

Treatment (n)	ASAS 20/40 responders	Partial remission	Patient global change (0–10 VAS)	Change in BASDAI	Change in BASFI
Infliximab 5 mg/kg (201)	61.2%/47%*	22.4%*	+49.7*	−2.9*	−1.7*
Placebo (78)	19.2%/12%	1.3%	+6.1	−0.4	0.0

*P < 0.001 vs placebo.

ASSERT week 24

Treatment (n)	Night pain (0–10 VAS)	Change in SF36, physical component	Change in BASMI	BASDAI 50
Infliximab 5 mg/kg (201)	−2.9*	10.2*	−1.0†	51%*
Placebo (78)	−0.3	0.8	−0.0	10.7%

*P < 0.001, †P = 0.019 vs placebo.

Subgroup analysis of pretreatment CRP levels showed that patients with CRP level less than or equal to three times the upper limit of normal had ASAS 20 responses to infliximab of 46.3% (n=90), compared with 21.1% in placebo-treated patients (n=38) (P=0.007), whereas patients with baseline CRP levels more than three times the upper limit of normal showed ASAS 20 responses to infliximab of 74.5% (n=106), versus 17.5% in patients receiving placebo (n=40) (P<0.001).

Enthesitis score using the Mander Enthesitis Index (range 0–90, median baseline value 8.0) showed no improvement, but the enthesitis component of the BASDAI improved significantly at week 24 in the active therapy group (median improvement 2.9) compared with placebo (worsening 0.2) (P<0.001).

MRI activity scores of spinal disease were improved in patients receiving infliximab versus placebo (P<0.001). The change in MRI chronicity scores was not significantly different in either group.

Bone density assessed by dual X-ray absorptiometry (DEXA) of the spine and hip improved significantly in the infliximab-treated group compared with placebo by week 24.

Treatment was continued for up to 102 weeks, with all patients receiving open-label infliximab 5 mg/kg every 6 weeks after week 24. ASAS 20 responses and other measures of improvement were maintained in those continuing infliximab and in those beginning after week 24, with both groups reaching and maintaining similar levels of improvement. From week 36 to 96, patients in the original active therapy group who had a BASDAI score >3 on two consecutive visits were able to dose escalate to 7.5 mg/kg. There was an increase in the numbers who achieved an ASAS 20 response, but this did not reach the same levels as those who maintained 5-mg/kg doses throughout the study period.

At week 102 the improvement from baseline of MRI activity scores seen at week 24 was maintained, and also achieved in the group switching from placebo.

DEXA bone density values continued to improve from week 24 to week 102. Scores in the group switching from placebo to infliximab were then similar to those in patients receiving infliximab for the total 102 weeks.

References

1 Elliott MJ, Maini RN, Feldmann M, et al. Treatment of rheumatoid arthritis with chimeric monoclonal antibodies to tumor necrosis factor alpha. *Arthritis Rheum* 1993; **36**: 1681–90.
2 Elliott MJ, Maini RN, Feldmann M, et al. Randomised double-blind comparison of chimeric monoclonal antibody to tumour necrosis factor alpha (cA2) versus placebo in rheumatoid arthritis. *Lancet* 1994; **344**: 1105–10.
3 Maini R, St Clair EW, Breedveld F, et al. Infliximab (chimeric anti-tumour necrosis factor alpha monoclonal antibody) versus placebo in rheumatoid arthritis patients receiving concomitant methotrexate: a randomised phase III trial. ATTRACT Study Group. *Lancet* 1999; **354**: 1932–9.
4 St Clair EW, Wagner CL, Fasanmade AA, et al. The relationship of serum infliximab concentrations to clinical improvement in rheumatoid arthritis: results from ATTRACT, a multicenter, randomised, double-blind, placebo-controlled trial. *Arthritis Rheum* 2002; **46**: 1451–9.
5 St Clair EW, van der Heijde DM, Smolen JS, et al.; Active-Controlled Study of Patients Receiving Infliximab for the Treatment of Rheumatoid Arthritis of Early Onset Study Group. Combination of infliximab and methotrexate therapy for early rheumatoid arthritis: a randomized, controlled trial. *Arthritis Rheum* 2004; **50**: 3432–43.
6 Westhovens R, Yocum D, Han J, et al. The safety of infliximab, combined with background treatments, among patients with rheumatoid arthritis and various comorbidities: a large, randomized, placebo-controlled trial. *Arthritis Rheum* 2006; **54**: 1075–86.
7 Antoni CE, Kavanaugh A, Kirkham B, et al. Sustained benefits of infliximab therapy for dermatologic and articular manifestations of psoriatic arthritis: results from the infliximab multinational psoriatic arthritis controlled trial (IMPACT). *Arthritis Rheum* 2005; **52**: 1227–36.
8 Kavanaugh A, Antoni CE, Gladman D, et al. The Infliximab Multinational Psoriatic Arthritis Controlled Trial (IMPACT): results of radiographic analyses after 1 year. *Ann Rheum Dis* 2006; **65**: 1038–43.
9 Antoni C, Krueger GG, de Vlam K, et al. Infliximab improves signs and symptoms of psoriatic arthritis: results of the IMPACT 2 trial. *Ann Rheum Dis* 2005; **64**: 1150–7.

10 Braun J, Brandt J, Listing J, *et al.* Treatment of active ankylosing spondylitis with infliximab: a randomised controlled multicentre trial. *Lancet* 2002; **359**: 1187–93.
11 van der Heijde D, Dijkmans B, Geusens P, *et al.*; Ankylosing Spondylitis Study for the Evaluation of Recombinant Infliximab Therapy Study Group. Efficacy and safety of infliximab in patients with ankylosing spondylitis: results of a randomized, placebo-controlled trial (ASSERT). *Arthritis Rheum* 2005; **52**: 582–91.

Certolizumab pegol (Cimzia)

Chemical properties	Pegylated humanized Fab′ fragment (95% human)
Manufacture	Expressed in *Escherichia coli*
Pharmacokinetics	Half-life is 14 days. It is administered subcutaneously and the interval between injections in the pivotal clinical trials was 2–4 weeks
Metabolism	Unclear; however, pegylation is responsible for a prolonged half-life compared to a non-pegylated Fab′ fragment
Drug interactions	Unclear. Azathioprine, 6-mercaptopurine, and MTX probably decrease the clearance rate

Clinical trial data – rheumatoid arthritis

Phase II and Rapid I [1,2] This study and preceding studies in RA used a lyophilized preparation. This preparation was changed to a liquid preparation (for use in prefilled syringes), which will be the licensed product for RA.

Rapid 2 – Phase III [3,4] Randomized double-blind study of liquid certolizumab pegol; 24-week study. Patients with active RA, mean age 52 years, mean disease duration 6 years, mean DAS28 6.8. Randomized 2:2:1, placebo, 200 mg s.c. every 2 weeks, after loading dose of 400 mg at weeks 0, 2, and 4, or 400 mg every 2 weeks. Patients who did not achieve an ACR 20 response at week 16 were withdrawn at week 12 or 14, classified as non-responders and data (last observation carried forward, LOCF) to week 24.

Rapid II

Dose (*n*)	ACR 20	ACR 50	ACR 70	Change in HAQ-DI	Patients achieving HAQ MCID	Change in mean X-ray progress*
200 mg e.o.w. (246)	57%†	32%†	16%‡	−0.50†	57%	−0.4
400 mg e.o.w. (246)	58%†	33%†	11%‡	−0.51†	53%	0.2
Placebo (127)	3%	8%	1%	−0.14	11%	1.3

e.o.w., every other week. MCID, minimum clinically important difference (0.22).
*Total van der Heijde/Sharp score.
†$P < 0.001$, ‡$P \leq 0.008$.

Safety Injection site pain reported in only one patient in the 400-mg group. Serious adverse events were infection: 20.8%, 27.8%, and 21.5% in the placebo, 200-mg and 400-mg groups, respectively. Likewise serious infections increased in the active therapy groups, placebo 0%, 3.2%, 2.4%. Most common serious infections were erysipelas, sinusitis, and TB. One death occurred in each of the active therapy arms.

References

1 Choy EH, Hazleman B, Smith M, *et al*. Efficacy of a novel PEGylated humanized anti-TNF fragment (CDP870) in patients with rheumatoid arthritis: a phase II double-blinded, randomized, dose-escalating trial. *Rheumatology (Oxford)* 2002; **41**:1133–7.
2 van der Heijde D, Strand V, Keystone E, and Landewe R. Inhibition of radiographic progression by lyophilised certolizumab pegol added to methotrexate in comparison to methotrexate alone in patients with rheumatoid arthritis: The Rapid 1 trial. *Arthritis Rheum* 2007; **56**: S390, ACR Meeting (Abstract No. 940).
3 Mease P, Mason D, Kavanaugh A, and Smolen J. Efficacy and rapid response of certolizumab pegol liquid formulation in combination with methotrexate in patients with active rheumatoid arthritis despite methotrexate therapy: results from RAPID 2. *Arthritis Rheum* 2007; **56**: S391, ACR Meeting (Abstract No. 941).
4 Landewe R, Strand V, Smolen J, and van der Heijde D. Liquid formulation certolizumab pegol with methotrexate decreases progression of structural joint damage in rheumatoid arthritis patients: The Rapid 2 trial. *Arthritis Rheum* 2007; **56**: S298, ACR Meeting (Abstract No. 696).

Abatacept (Orencia)

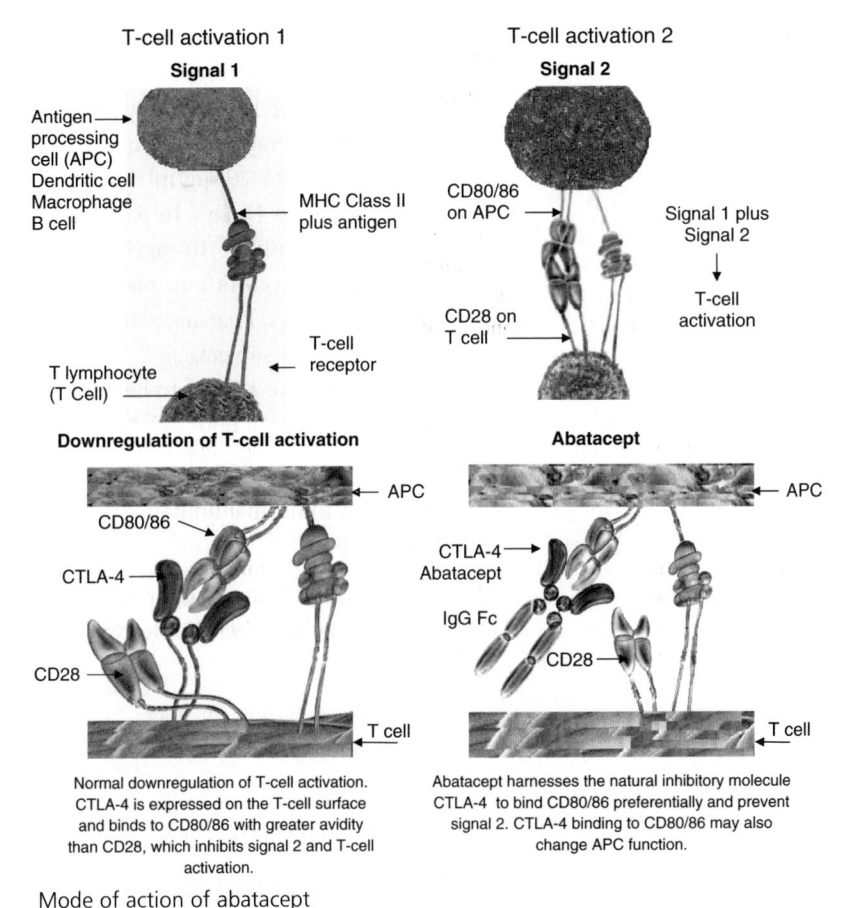

T-cell activation 1
Signal 1

Antigen processing cell (APC) Dendritic cell Macrophage B cell

MHC Class II plus antigen

T lymphocyte (T Cell)

T-cell receptor

T-cell activation 2
Signal 2

CD80/86 on APC

CD28 on T cell

Signal 1 plus Signal 2
↓
T-cell activation

Downregulation of T-cell activation

APC
CD80/86
CTLA-4
CD28
T cell

Normal downregulation of T-cell activation. CTLA-4 is expressed on the T-cell surface and binds to CD80/86 with greater avidity than CD28, which inhibits signal 2 and T-cell activation.

Abatacept

APC
CTLA-4 Abatacept
IgG Fc
CD28
T cell

Abatacept harnesses the natural inhibitory molecule CTLA-4 to bind CD80/86 preferentially and prevent signal 2. CTLA-4 binding to CD80/86 may also change APC function.

Mode of action of abatacept

Chemical properties	Recombinant fusion protein made from the extracellular domain of human cytotoxic T-lymphocyte-associated antigen 4 (CTLA-4) linked to modified Fc chain of human IgG1, 92-kDa
	CTLA-4 binds 4-fold less avidly to CD86 than to CD80
Manufacture	Produced in a mammalian cell expression system

Stability	Supplied as a lyophilized powder stable if stored in the dark at 2–8°C
Pharmacokinetics	After a 10-mg/kg single intravenous infusion in healthy volunteers or infusions on days 1, 15, 30, and then monthly, in patients with RA, average peak serum concentration was 292–295 μg/ml. Half-life is between 13 and 17 days. In patients with RA receiving multiple 10-mg/kg infusions, serum concentrations reached steady state by 60 days. Pharmacokinetics are similar in healthy subjects and patients with RA, with a trend to higher clearance with increased bodyweight
Metabolism	Unclear, but thought to be catabolized in a similar manner to normal human immunoglobulin
Drug interactions	MTX, NSAIDs, corticosteroids, or TNF-blocking drugs do not alter the clearance of abatacept
Dosage	Approximately 10 mg/kg, given as an intravenous infusion over 30 min
	Weight <60 kg: 500 mg (two vials)
	Weight 60–100 kg: 750 mg (three vials)
	Weight >100 kg: 1000 mg (four vials)

Clinical trial data – rheumatoid arthritis

Phase I studies investigated intravenous abatacept in doses ranging from 0.5 to 10 mg/kg.

Phase II/III studies

The main outcomes measures for these studies were the American College of Rheumatology response criteria (ACR 20/50/70), denoting an improvement of at least 20%, 50%, or 70% of RA activity. These studies were performed in the USA and worldwide, and are summarized below.

Study I – USA, Phase II [1] Abatacept monotherapy versus placebo for 8 weeks. 122 patients failing at least one DMARD or etanercept, mean disease duration approximately 3.7 years.

Study I

Dose (*n*)	ACR 20	ACR 50	ACR 70
0.5 mg/kg (26)	23%	0%	0%
2.0 mg/kg (32)	44%	19%	12%
10 mg/kg (32)	53%	16%	6%
Placebo (32)	31%	6%	0%

*$P < 0.05$ vs placebo.

Study II – USA, Argentina, Europe, Australia, Canada, Phase IIb [2] 12-month study, data analysis at 6 and 12 months. Patients not responding to MTX, average dose in active therapy group 15.4 mg, placebo group 15.8 mg/week. Mean age 55 years, 68% female, mean disease duration 9.3 years.

Study II: 6-month data

Dose (*n*)	ACR 20	ACR 50	ACR 70
2 mg/kg (105)	42%	23%*	11%*
10 mg/kg (115)	60%*	37%*	17%*
Placebo (119)	35%	12%	2%

*$P < 0.05$ vs placebo.

Study II: 12-month data

Dose (*n*)	ACR 20	ACR 50	ACR 70	Change in M-HAQ	Remission (DAS28 <2.6)
2 mg/kg (105)	40%	22%	12%	−23%	22%
10 mg/kg (115)	63%*	42%*	21%*	−42%*	35%*
Placebo (119)	36%	20%	8%	−10%	10%

*$P < 0.05$ vs placebo.

AIM Study – worldwide, Phase III [3,4] 12-month study. Patients not responding to MTX, average dose in active therapy group 16.1 mg/week, placebo group 15.7 mg/week. Mean age 51 years, 80% female, mean disease duration 8.7 years.

AIM Study

Dose (n)	ACR 20	ACR 50	ACR 70	Change in HAQ-DI	Remission (DAS28 <2.6)
10 mg/kg (433)	73%*	48%*	29%*	−0.68*	24%*
Placebo (219)	40%	18%	6%	−0.50	2%

*$P < 0.05$ vs placebo.

ATTAIN Study – worldwide, Phase III [5] Failed previous TNF-blocker therapy, 40% currently, 60% formerly; etanercept 35%, infliximab 65%, adalimumab 2%. Mean age 53 years, 78% female. Abatacept group, 76% on MTX, 15 mg/week; placebo, 82% on MTX, 14 mg/week. Outcomes at 6 months, remission defined by Disease Activity Score (DAS28) <2.6.

ATTAIN

Dose (n)	ACR 20	ACR 50	ACR 70	Remission	Change in HAQ-DI
10 mg/kg approx. (258)	50%*	20%*	10%*	10%*	−0.45*
Placebo (133)	20%	4%	2%	1%	−0.11

*$P < 0.05$ vs placebo.

ASSURE Study – USA, Europe, Phase III [6] One-year safety study of abatacept (10 mg/kg approx.) versus placebo with continuing non-biologic DMARDs including MTX, sulfasalazine, leflunomide, intramuscular gold, and hydroxychloroquine/chloroquine, and biologic DMARDs, etanercept 64%, infliximab 19%, adalimumab 11%, anakinra 13%.

ASSURE

Treatment (n)	Serious infections	Change in HAQ-DI	Patient global
Abatacept/DMARD (856)	2.6%	−0.47	−41%
Placebo/DMARD (418)	1.7%	−0.26	−20%
Abatacept/biologic DMARD (103)	5.8%	−0.33	−36%
Placebo/biologic DMARD (86)	1.6%	−0.23	−28%

ATTEST study – USA, South America, South Africa, Mexico, France [7] Evaluation of abatacept or infliximab versus placebo. Patients with RA with an inadequate response to MTX, average dose 16.5 mg/week, randomized 3:3:2, to abatacept (approx. 10 mg/kg every 4 weeks), infliximab (3 mg/kg usual regimen), or placebo infusions in a double-blind double-dummy controlled study. To ensure blinding to treatment group assignment, patients received two infusions on the day of treatment, one over 30min (abatacept or placebo) and the other over 2 hours (infliximab or placebo). Primary outcome was mean change in DAS28 for abatacept versus placebo at day 197.

ATTEST

Treatment (n)	ACR 20	ACR 50	ACR 70	Remission	Change in DAS28	HAQ (% MCID)
Abatacept 10mg/kg (156)						
Day 197 approx. (139)	66.7%*	40.4%*	20.5%	11.3%	−2.53*	61.5%*
Day 365	72.4%	45.5%	26.3%	18.7%	−2.88	40.9%
Placebo (110), day 197	41.8%	20%	9.1%	2.9%	−1.48	

MCID, minimum clinically important difference.
*P<0.001, †P=0.019 vs placebo.

ATTEST

Treatment (n)	ACR 20	ACR 50	ACR 70	Remission	Change in DAS28	HAQ (% MCID)
Infliximab 3mg/kg						
Day 197 (165)	59.4%*	37.0%†	24.2%‡	12.8%	−2.23§	58.8%#
Day 365 (141)	55.8%	36.4%	20.6%	12.2%	−2.25	40.9%
Placebo (110), day 197	41.8%	20%	9.1%	2.9%	−1.48	

*P<0.006, †P=0.004, ‡P=0.002, §P< 0.001, #P=0.005 vs placebo.

Changes in DAS scores were similar for abatacept and infliximab at day 197, but greater in the abatacept group at day 365 (χ^2 test and confidence intervals employed). ACR 50 and 70 responses were not significantly different at 12 months.

Adverse events were similar in all groups up to day 197, although the inflixiamb group had a higher proportion of related serious adverse events compared with placebo (4.8% vs 2.7%) and discontinuation due to serious adverse effects (SAEs) (2.4% vs 0%). This difference consisted largely of serious infections. Infusion reactions occurred in 5.1% of patients receiving abatacept, 10.8% of those receiving placebo, and 18.2% receiving infliximab.

Infectious adverse events over the 12-month study period were higher in the infliximab-treated group than in the abatacept-treated group: serious infections 8.5% versus 1.9%; discontinuations due to SAEs 3.6% versus 2.6%.

The conclusion of these studies is that abatacept is efficacious as monotherapy, and that the combination with MTX and most other DMARDs is safe. However, the combination of abatacept with other biological DMARDs (TNF-blockers and anakinra) is associated with a significant increase in serious infections and is not recommended. Abatacept significantly reduces progression of radiological joint damage in patients with RA. The efficacy of abatacept in patients with early RA is not known.

Safety of abatacept

Safety data reported here are derived from the clinical trial programme reported to the US Food and Drug Administration (FDA), which enrolled 1955 patients treated with abatacept and 989 treated with placebo (abatacept at 1 year, 1697; placebo at 1 year, 856).

Infection

In the clinical trial programme, the most commonly reported infections resulting in dose interruption in patients receiving abatacept were upper respiratory tract infections (1.0%), bronchitis (0.7%), and herpes zoster (0.7%). The most frequent infections causing dose discontinuation were pneumonia (0.2%), localized infections (0.2%), and bronchitis (0.1%).

Serious infections were reported in 3.0% of patients receiving abatacept compared with 1.9% of those receiving placebo, the most common being pneumonia, cellulitis, urinary tract infections, bronchitis, diverticulitis, and acute pyelonephritis.

Patients in studies were screened for latent TB, and no experience has been gained of using abatacept in patients with this condition. It is recommended that all patients should be screened for latent TB, using similar protocols as for TNF-blocker drugs.

A subset of 37 patients with chronic obstructive pulmonary disease (COPD) received abatacept (20) or placebo (17). In this group more patients receiving abatacept reported serious adverse events than for placebo (24% vs 6%. respectively), including exacerbations of COPD (8%) and pneumonia (2%).

Malignancy

In the placebo-controlled study periods, the frequencies of malignancy were similar for patients receiving abatacept and placebo (1.3% vs 1.1%). However, more cases of lung cancer were observed in the abatacept group (four patients;

0.2% vs 0%). The cumulative trial data, including placebo-controlled and uncontrolled studies (2688 patients, 3827 patient-years), reported eight cases of lung cancer (0.21 per 100 patient-years) and four cases of lymphoma (0.1 per 100 patient-years). The lymphoma rate was 3.5-fold higher than the age- and sex-matched general population (SEER [Surveillance Epidemiology and End Results] database), compatible with rates seen in patients with active RA.

Infusion and hypersensitivity reactions

Acute infusion reactions (occurring within 1 hour of infusion) were noted in 9% of patients receiving abatacept compared with 6% receiving placebo. Most were mild, mainly dizziness, headache, and hypertension. Less common events (<1%, >0.1%) included hypotension, hypertension, dyspnoea, nausea, flushing, and urticaria. Most were mild to moderate. Less than 1% of patients receiving abatacept discontinued studies because of infusion reactions (six vs two on placebo). In 2688 patients receiving abatacept, only two cases of anaphylaxis were reported.

Blood glucose monitoring

Parenteral products containing maltose, such as abatacept, can interfere with blood glucose reading strips that contain glucose dehydrogenase pyrroloquinolonequinone (GDH-PQQ). The interference can give falsely raised readings. Patients taking abatacept are advised to use alternative methods, utilizing other reactions such as GDH-NAD, glucose oxidase, or glucose hexokinase.

Immunogenicity

Anti-abatacept antibodies were found in 1.7% of patients (34 of 1993) during therapy, increasing to 5.8% after drug had cleared from serum; six of nine tested were neutralizing, although there was no correlation with clinical outcomes or adverse events.

Pregnancy and lactation

Abatacept is classified as Class C as there are no data from human trials of pregnant women receiving the drug. Animal studies have shown no teratogenic potential. There was a suggestion of an increased autoimmune response in rat pups. The drug was found to be excreted in rat milk.

References

1 Moreland LW, Alten R, Van den Bosch F, *et al*. Costimulatory blockade in patients with rheumatoid arthritis: a pilot, dose-finding, double-blind, placebo-controlled clinical trial evaluating CTLA-4Ig and LEA29Y eighty-five days after the first infusion. *Arthritis Rheum* 2002; **46**: 1470–9.

2 Kremer JM, Westhovens R, Leon M, *et al.* Treatment of rheumatoid arthritis by selective inhibition of T-cell activation with fusion protein CTLA4Ig. *N Engl J Med* 2003; **349**: 1907–15.

3 Kremer JM, Dougados M, Emery P, *et al.* Treatment of rheumatoid arthritis with the selective costimulation modulator abatacept: twelve-month results of a phase IIb, double-blind, randomized, placebo-controlled trial. *Arthritis Rheum* 2005; **52**: 2263–71.

4 Kremer JM, Genant HK, Moreland LW, *et al.* Effects of abatacept in patients with methotrexate-resistant active rheumatoid arthritis: a randomized trial. *Ann Intern Med* 2006; **144**: 865–76.

5 Genovese MC, Becker J-C, Schiff M, *et al.* Abatacept for rheumatoid arthritis refractory to tumor necrosis factor α inhibition. *N Engl J Med* 2005; **353**: 1114–23.

6 Weinblatt M, Combe B, White A, *et al.* Safety of abatacept in patients with active rheumatoid arthritis receiving background non-biologic and biologic DMARDs: 1-year results of the ASSURE trial. *Ann Rheum Dis* 2005; **64**(Suppl III): 60.

7 Schiff M, Keiserman M, Codding C, *et al.* Efficacy and safety of abatacept or infliximab versus placebo in ATTEST: a phase III, multicenter, randomized, double-blind, placebo-controlled study in patients with rheumatoid arthritis and an inadequate response to methotrexate. *Ann Rheum Dis* 2007 [Epub ahead of print].

Anakinra (Kineret)

Chemical properties	Recombinant non-glycosylated form of the human interleukin-1 receptor antagonist (IL-1Ra), identical to native human IL-1Ra apart from a methionine residue added to the amino terminus (r-metHuIL-1Ra). Recommended daily dose for RA is 100 mg daily
Manufacture	Produced in an *E. coli* expression system
Stability	Stable for 18 months if stored in the dark at 2–8°C. May be removed once from cool storage for a maximum of 12 hours in temperatures up to 25°C
Pharmacokinetics	Anakinra is well absorbed after subcutaneous injection, with bioavailability of a 70-mg bolus injection in healthy subjects of 95%. In subjects with RA, maximum plasma concentrations are reached 3–7 hours after subcutaneous injection of 1–2-mg/kg doses. Terminal half-life is 4–6 hours. Sex and age do not significantly reduce clearance of anakinra. No safety signals have been observed in clinical trials in patients older than 65 years, compared with patients of younger age. Pharmacokinetics are similar in healthy subjects and patients with RA
Metabolism	Anakinra clearance correlates with creatinine clearance and body weight. Mean plasma clearance decreased by 70–75% in patients with severe and end-stage renal failure. Caution required if used in patients with moderate renal dysfunction (Cl_{cr} 30–50 ml/min). Not recommended in patients with severe renal failure (Cl_{cr} <30 ml/min). No dose adjustment required in hepatic impairment
Drug interactions	DMARD, NSAID, and corticosteroid interactions have not been formally investigated, but in clinical trials do not have any detectable interactions with anakinra. No interaction of MTX and anakinra in rats

Clinical trial data – rheumatoid arthritis

Phase II dose-ranging study [1] Patients in nine different dosing groups were treated for an initial 3 weeks with interleukin (IL)-1ra either 20, 70, or 200 mg weekly, three times per week or daily, followed by a 4-week maintenance phase, receiving the starting dose once per week. This study showed that daily dosing was superior to less frequent dosing regimens.

Study I – Phase II monotherapy study, Europe [2,3] Placebo-controlled, 24-week study. Patients with active RA of duration >6 months and <8 years, mean age 53 years, 75% female, 69% RF-positive, mean disease duration 4 years, mean SJC 26, TJC 34, ESR 50 mm/hour, CRP 4 mg/dl. Four groups: placebo or IL-1ra at either 30, 75, or 150 mg daily by subcutaenous injection. DMARDs discontinued at least 6 weeks prior to enrolment.

Monotherapy study

Dose (*n*)	ACR 20	ACR 50	ACR 70	Change in HAQ	Change in total Sharp score (week 48)*	Change in CRP (mg/dl)
30 mg daily (119)	39%			−0.2†	1.5	−1.3
75 mg daily (116)	34%	11%	1%	−0.2†	1.7*	−1.0
150 mg daily (116)	43%†	19%†	1%	−0.3‡	1.5*	−1.0
Placebo (119)	27%	8%	1%	−0.04	3.4	−0.4

*Reduction of joint space narrowing was greater than erosion score.

†$P < 0.05$, ‡$P < 0.01$ vs placebo.

Study 2 – USA, Australia, Canada, Phase III [4] 24-week study. Patients not responding to MTX, average dose 17 mg/week. Mean age 53 years, 76% female, disease duration 7 years. Six treatment groups, intention-to-treat analysis.

Study 2

Dose (*n*)	ACR 20	ACR 50	ACR 70	Change in HAQ	Change in CRP (mg/dl)
0.04 mg/kg/day (63)	19%	13%	5%		
0.1 mg/kg/day (74)	30%	20%	7%		
0.4 mg/kg/day (77)	36%	11%	2%		
1.0 mg/kg/day (59)	42%*	24%*	10%*	−0.37*	−0.77
2.0 mg/kg/day (72)	35%	17%	7%	−0.51†	−0.77
Placebo (74)	23%	4%	0%	−0.15	−0.19

*$P < 0.05$, †$P < 0.0005$ vs placebo.

Confirmatory efficacy study [5] Placebo-controlled study of anakinra 100 mg/day in combination with MTX, versus placebo. Patients not responding to MTX, average dose ranging from 16.3 to 17.6 mg/week. Age range 49–54 years, 63–85% female, disease duration 6.3–8.8 years, intention-to-treat analysis, weeks 12 and 24.

Confirmatory study: week 24

Dose (n)	ACR 20	ACR 50	ACR 70	Change in HAQ	Change in CRP (mg/dl)
100 mg (250)	38%*	17%†	6%*	−0.29*	−1.7*
Placebo (251)	22%	8%	2%	−0.18	−0.6

*$P < 0.05$, †$P < 0.001$ vs placebo.

Safety of anakinra

The most common adverse event was injection site reactions, which occurred in 71% of patients receiving anakinra, compared with 28% of patients receiving placebo injections. Most reactions were mild, characterized as erythema, ecchymosis, inflammation, and/or pain, leading to study withdrawal in 5.6% of patients. Most reactions occurred within the first 4 weeks of therapy and median duration was 14–28 days.

Serious infections were slightly increased compared with placebo (1.8% vs 0.7%, respectively), mainly bacterial infections, cellulitis, pneumonia, bone and joint infections. No cases of TB or opportunistic infection were reported. Neutropenia was reported in 2.4% of patients receiving anakinra versus 0.4% of controls. It is recommended to check neutrophil count monthly for the first 6 months of anakinra therapy. No deaths were reported in the clinical trial programme.

Long-term safety seems to be similar to that reported in the placebo-controlled components of studies. No increase in malignancy compared with rates in the SEER database were reported [6,7].

References

1. Campion GV, Lebsack ME, Lookabaugh J, Gordon G, Catalano M; The IL-1Ra Arthritis Study Group. Dose-range and dose-frequency study of recombinant human interleukin-1 receptor antagonist in patients with rheumatoid arthritis. *Arthritis Rheum* 1996; **39**: 1092–101.
2. Bresnihan B, Alvaro-Gracia JM, Cobby M, *et al*. Treatment of rheumatoid arthritis with recombinant human interleukin-1 receptor antagonist. *Arthritis Rheum* 1998; **41**: 2196–204.

3. Bresnihan B, Newmark R, Robbins S, and Genant HK. Effects of anakinra monotherapy on joint damage in patients with rheumatoid arthritis. Extension of a 24-week randomized, placebo-controlled trial. *J Rheumatol* 2004; **31**: 1103–11.
4. Cohen S, Hurd E, Cush J, *et al.* Treatment of rheumatoid arthritis with anakinra, a recombinant human interleukin-1 receptor antagonist, in combination with methotrexate: results of a twenty-four-week, multicenter, randomized, double-blind, placebo-controlled trial. *Arthritis Rheum* 2002; **46**: 614–24.
5. Cohen SB, Moreland LW, Cush JJ, *et al.*; 990145 Study Group. A multicentre, double blind, randomised, placebo controlled trial of anakinra (Kineret), a recombinant interleukin 1 receptor antagonist, in patients with rheumatoid arthritis treated with background methotrexate. *Ann Rheum Dis* 2004; **63**: 1062–8.
6. Fleischmann RM, Schechtman J, Bennett R, *et al.* Anakinra, a recombinant human interleukin-1 receptor antagonist (r-metHuIL-1ra), in patients with rheumatoid arthritis: a large, international, multicenter, placebo-controlled trial. *Arthritis Rheum* 2003; **48**: 927–34.
7. Fleischmann RM, Tesser J, Schiff MH, *et al.* Safety of extended treatment with anakinra in patients with rheumatoid arthritis. *Ann Rheum Dis* 2006; **65**: 1006–12.

B-cell depletion: Rituximab (Rituxan® [USA], MabThera® [Europe, Asia, South America])

Chemical properties	Chimaeric IgG1 ? monoclonal antibody (145 kDa)
Manufacture	Produced in Chinese Hamster Ovary (CHO) cells
Stability	Stable when stored at 2–8°C (36–46°F). Not to be used after expiration date on carton. Should be protected from direct sunlight. Should not be frozen or shaken. Supplied as 100- and 500-mg sterile, preservative-free, single-use vials
Pharmacokinetics	The pharmacokinetics of rituximab as used in autoimmune disease may differ from those in non-Hodgkin's lymphoma, owing to differences in the number of CD20+ cells and possibly other factors. In patients with RA, after the administration of two doses of rituximab, the mean C_{max} values were 183 µg/ml for the 2 × 500-mg dose and 370 µg/ml for the 2 × 1000-mg dose. Following the 2 × 1000-mg rituximab dose, the mean volume of distribution at steady state was 4.3 litres (CV = 28%), suggesting largely intravascular distribution. Mean systemic serum clearance of rituximab was 0.01 litres/hour, and mean terminal elimination half-life after the second dose was 19 days
Mechanism	CD20 is a lineage-specific B-cell marker that is present from the pre-B cell stage through to mature B cells, being absent on stem cells and plasma cells. Treatment with rituximab leads to depletion of CD20-expressing cells by mechanisms including complement-mediated lysis, antibody-dependent cellular cytotoxicity, and induction of apoptosis
Metabolism	As with other therapeutic monoclonal antibodies, rituximab is thought to be processed in a similar manner to normal immunoglobulin (IgG)
Drug interactions	In RA, the concomitant use of MTX does not appear to affect the clearance of rituximab

Clinical trial data – rheumatoid arthritis

Rituximab was initially studied and approved (in 1997) for the treatment of patients with non-Hodgkin's lymphoma (NHL).

Phase I studies in RA suggested the potential efficacy of B-cell depletion in that condition. The dose regimens were based loosely on those previously used in NHL. However, rather than 4-weekly injections of 375 mg/m^2, two doses of 1000 mg were given at a 2-week interval. In the early studies, many patients received concomitant therapy with cyclophosphamide and high-dose corticosteroids. Most patients had positive tests for serum RF.

Phase II/III studies A phase II study in RF-positive patients with RA and active disease, despite concomitant use of MTX, evaluated the effect of rituximab monotherapy, or rituximab in combination with MTX or cyclophosphamide, and compared this with MTX monotherapy [1]. All patients received methylprednisolone given intravenously before infusions and orally between infusions, with a total dose of approximately 700 mg. Rituximab was given as two infusions of 1000 mg each on days 1 and 15. Cyclophosphamide was given at a dose of 750 mg intravenously on days 3 and 17.

Patients receiving rituximab experienced higher levels of response than those receiving MTX monotherapy. Combination therapy with cyclophosphamide, and particularly with MTX, appeared to prolong the duration of response.

Phase II study: treatment responses at 24 weeks [1]

Treatment (*n*)	ACR 20	ACR 50	ACR 70
MTX (40)	38%	13%	5%
Rituximab (40)	65%*	33%*	15%
Rituximab + MTX (40)	73%*	43%*	23%*
Rituximab + cyclophosphamide (41)	76%*	41%*	15%

*$P < 0.05$ vs MTX group.

DANCER – Phase II study [2] A subsequent phase II study (known as DANCER) evaluated several doses of rituximab and also of peri-infusional corticosteroids in patients with active RA despite the concomitant use of MTX [2]. Previous treatment with TNF inhibitors was allowed, and about 31% of patients had received such therapy. A subset of RF-negative patients was enrolled. Patients remained on stable MTX, and were randomized to receive two infusions of placebo, rituximab 500 mg, or rituximab 1000 mg on days 1 and 15. In addition, patients were randomized to receive no corticosteroids, intravenous methylprednisolone pre-infusion, or intravenous methylprednisolone pre-infusion, as well as oral steroids between infusions.

Treatment was effective, and there was no significant difference between rituximab doses. Overall, the use of steroids did not affect efficacy. Patients receiving steroids did experience a slight reduction in infusion reactions to the first dose of rituximab.

DANCER: 24 weeks

Treatment (*n*)	ACR 20	ACR 50	ACR 70
Rituximab 500 mg (123)	55%*	33%*	13%*
Rituximab 1000 mg (122)	54%*	34%*	20%*
Placebo (122)	28%	13%	5%

*$P < 0.05$ vs placebo.

REFLEX – Phase II study [3] The pivotal phase II study (known as REFLEX) evaluated the efficacy of rituximab in patients who had failed previous therapy with one or more TNF inhibitors [3]. Patients received 1000 mg rituximab on days 1 and 15, and corticosteroids pre-infusion and between infusions. Efficacy was established in this population.

REFLEX: 24 weeks

Treatment (*n*)	ACR 20	ACR 50	ACR 70
Rituximab (298)	51%*	27%*	12%*
Placebo (201)	18%	5%	1%

*$P < 0.0001$ vs placebo.

Subanalysis data from this study suggested that the extent of responses may be greater among patients who are RF positive or who have antibodies to cyclic citrullinated peptide (CCP) than in those who are seronegative to both.

Analysis of radiographs at 1 year showed a significant effect of rituximab therapy in inhibiting the progression of radiological damage. This benefit appeared to be independent of the extent of clinical response.

The conclusion of these studies is that rituximab is effective as a therapy for RA. Patients who have failed previous therapy with TNF inhibitors respond significantly, as do those who have not received such therapy.

Frequently asked questions

What about safety?

There are a number of safety considerations related to the use of rituximab. As noted, rituximab has been approved for use in NHL since 1997; therefore, there is a relatively large and longstanding database from which to draw longer-term safety information and pharmacovigilance data surrounding this drug.

Infusion reactions With intravenous administration of rituximab, infusion reactions have been observed. In some cases these have been serious, even fatal. The most severe reactions tend to occur with the first administration. It appears than infusion reactions may be both more common and more severe in NHL than in RA. In part, this may be explained by the potential occurrence of tumour lysis syndrome in patients with NHL, particularly those with a large tumour burden of CD20+ cells.

Infections As with any immunomodulatory agent, there is the potential for rituximab to interfere with normal immune function and thereby predispose to infections. In clinical studies of RA, a higher incidence of infections, but not of serious infections, was seen with treatment. There are several particular concerns regarding viral infection with rituximab. Fatal cases of reactivation of hepatitis B have been observed, and screening for hepatitis B virus should be done before treatment. A number of other viral infections, representing new infections, reactivations, or exacerbations, have also been observed, so clinicians should be alert to symptoms suggestive of infection. In NHL and in several patients with systemic lupus erythematosus, cases of progressive multifocal leucoencephalopathy (PML), many of which were fatal, have been observed.

Pregnancy In animal models, administration of rituximab affected the development of lymphoid tissue in the offspring. Therefore, rituximab is category 'C' as regards pregnancy. It is recommended that rituximab not be used by nursing mothers.

How should repeated doses of rituximab be given in RA?

In RA clinical studies, patients were allowed to enrol in long-term open-label extension follow-up with repeated treatments. Repeat courses of rituximab, often given at the same dose scheme, were typically administered when the disease activity had recurred. This ranged from 6 months after treatment (often the earliest timepoint allowed for retreatment) to 18–24 months or longer.

What about B-cell numbers?

Profound (e.g. >95% decrease) depletion of circulating B cells was observed in nearly all patients with RA after treatment with rituximab. Numbers of B cells began to return after several months in many, but not all, patients. Of note, there is no correlation between B-cell depletion and clinical response. Therefore, considerations for retreatment need to be made on clinical data.

Should immunoglobulin levels be measured?

In most patients with RA, treatment with a single course of rituximab resulted in a slight decrease in serum IgM levels. Decreases in IgG concentration occurred less commonly and to a lesser extent. With repeated courses, further changes in immunoglobulin levels may be expected, and it may be reasonable to measure quantitative immunoglobulins over time. Patients with immunoglobulin levels below the normal range were largely excluded from studies of RA.

What about using other therapies after rituximab?

There is limited information concerning the use of other antirheumatic therapies in patients with RA who have been treated with rituximab. A small series of patients (about 100) received TNF inhibitors after rituximab therapy, and it appears that such therapy was generally well tolerated.

Can rituximab be used in other rheumatic diseases?

Several large controlled clinical studies are under way assessing the use of rituximab in SLE. In the clinic, the use of rituximab in SLE is not uncommon. A number of other diseases are also under study, including those with clear autoantibody associations (e.g. antineutrophilic cytoplasmic antibodies [ANCA]-associated vasculitides), as well as conditions without such association (e.g. multiple sclerosis).

References

1 Edwards JCW, Szczepanski L, Szechinski J, et al. Efficacy of B-cell-targeted therapy with rituximab in patients with rheumatoid arthritis. *N Engl J Med* 2004; **350**: 2572–81.
2 Emery P, Fleischmann RM, Filipowicz-Sosnowska A, et al. The efficacy and safety of rituximab in patients with active rheumatoid arthritis despite methotrexate treatment: results of a phase IIb randomized trial. *Arthritis Rheum* 2006; **54**: 1390–400.
3 Cohen SB, Emery P, Greenwald MW, et al. Rituximab for rheumatoid arthritis refractory to anti-tumor necrosis factor therapy: results of a multicenter, randomized, double-blind, placebo-controlled, phase III trial evaluating primary efficacy and safety at twenty-four weeks. *Arthritis Rheum* 2006; **54**: 2793–806.

3
Dermatology

Psoriasis

Psoriasis is a common chronic skin disease for which great advances in terms of pathogenesis and treatment have been seen over the past few years. The term psoriasis embraces a spectrum of clinical disease with variation in phenotype, extent, and associated co-morbitities such as psoriatic arthritis [1]. Although typically thought of as being a 'benign disease', it is becoming increasingly apparent that a large number of diseases are associated with psoriasis and that the disease carries with it an excess mortality [2]. In addition, more patients, regardless of the severity of their condition, may suffer from a reduced quality of life, particularly as they relate to work and social and personal interactions [3].

Psoriasis affects approximately 2% of the general population, although prevalence is highly variable between races. It is thought to be most prevalent amongst white caucasians living in north Europe and Scandinavia. Several different phenotypic variants of psoriasis exist, including guttate psoriasis and pustular forms of the disease, but by far the commonest is psoriasis vulgaris (chronic plaque psoriasis), which accounts for 85–90% of all cases [4]. Virtually all trials of psoriasis relate to this latter phenotype. The usual age of onset is between 20 and 35 years of age with 75% of all cases occurring for the first time before the age of 46 years. Psoriasis vulgaris is characterized by the presence of well demarcated, indurated, red, scaly plaques. In mild cases these plaques are typically confined to extensor surfaces such as the elbows and knees, and also frequently involve the scalp and buttocks. The disease may spread to involve all of the skin (erythrodermic psoriasis). Symptoms range from nothing through pruritus to pain and soreness. Psoriasis can be extremely disfiguring. Widespread psoriasis can produce symptoms of general malaise. Between 5% and 25% of all cases of psoriasis are associated with a seronegative arthritis, termed psoriatic arthritis. Psoriasis, at least in moderate and severe forms, is associated with the metabolic syndrome (obesity, hyperinsulinaemia, hyperlipidaemia, hypertension) and also an increased morbidity and mortality associated with cardiovascular disease [5]. Debate exists about whether the disease is primarily associated with an increased risk of cancer, particularly lymphoma. Importantly, the disease is also associated with depressive illness and a higher rate of suicide.

In recent years there have been dramatic advances in our knowledge of the pathogenesis of psoriasis. It is clear that genes play an important role in pathogenesis. Approximately 30% of all patients give a history of an affected first-degree relative. Molecular genetic analysis reveals the presence of a major gene (as yet undetermined) within the major histocompatibility complex (MHC) on chromosome 6p. Genetic variation at this site is thought to account for between 35% and 50% of genetic susceptibility to psoriasis [6]. Progress has also been made in identifying genes of minor effect. Importantly, these provide major insight into relevant pathogenetic mechanisms. For example, functionally significant variation in the gene coding for the interleukin (IL)-23 receptor is associated with psoriasis [7,8]. Backed up by functional and clinical studies (see below), this has provided important clues into the precise immunological mechanisms involved in the disease.

Psoriasis is commonly regarded as an immune-mediated disease in which T helper 1 (Th1) cells play a critical role. Current evidence suggests that epidermal hyperproliferation, a cardinal feature of the disease, is driven by immunological mechanisms [9]. The advent of new biological therapies, particularly the effect of tumour necrosis factor (TNF) α-targeted therapy, has helped to reveal a critical role that innate immune responses play in disease pathogenesis. Thus, the pathogenic paradigm most often quoted suggests that, in genetically susceptible individuals, events occur that lead to activation of the innate immune system, which in turn, perhaps through IL-23-mediated mechanisms, leads to activation of the acquired immune system, and consequent epidermal hyperproliferation. Based on this new knowledge there has been an explosion of interest in psoriasis as a disease in which defined biological targets can lead to rapid resolution. Thus it appears that psoriasis is a good model of organ-specific autoimmune disease.

Approaches to management

Psoriasis treatment can be broadly subdivided into three categories: (a) topical treatment, (b) phototherapy, and (c) systemic therapy [1]. In general, standard practice is to start with topical therapy. If this is inadequate or there are problems, phototherapy is added. Finally systemic therapy is used when topical and phototherapy fail. Clearly this paradigm is dependent on the particular phenotype and extent of the disease. Topical treatment and phototherapy can be maximized in daycare facilities. In the UK, phototherapy and systemic therapy require referral to a dermatologist. Topical treatments are prescribed by general practitioners. It is estimated that between 20% and 30% of all patients with psoriasis will at some stage require either phototherapy or systemic therapy to control their disease (sometimes referred to as second-line therapy).

There are three licensed oral systemic therapies for psoriasis in Europe and the USA: methotrexate, ciclosporin, and acitretin. In Germany, fumaric acid esters are also licensed. Other oral drugs sometimes used to treat psoriasis include hydroxyurea, azathioprine, and mycophenolate. It is apparent that all of these drugs have significant side effects which limit their usage and also necessitate extensive monitoring. How to use them, and when they are best used, is beyond the scope of this book. Nevertheless it is important to remember that these drugs can be highly effective. In most countries, methotrexate remains the 'gold standard' for long-term treatment of severe psoriasis.

Assessing disease severity

Critical to the success of clinical trials in psoriasis assessing the efficacy of a therapeutic intervention is the use of validated assessment tools. A number of tools have been used in psoriasis clinical studies, indicating that debate exists amongst investigators as to which measure provides the best test. In practice, however, the primary efficacy variable utilized in the vast majority of studies (particularly pivotal studies) is the Psoriasis Area and Severity Index (PASI). This test provides a semiquantitative compound measurement of body surface area involved, degree of erythema, degree of scale, and degree of induration. The PASI does not take into account the effect of the psoriasis on the patient's quality of life. Hence, quality-of-life measures are frequently used as secondary variables. Of these, the most frequently used is the Dermatology Life Quality Index (DLQI).

Although the theoretical maximum PASI score is 72, by convention a PASI score greater than 10 is regarded as a measure of moderate disease. A PASI score above 20 is a measure of severe disease. Equally, a DLQI score (which can reach a maximum of 30) greater than 10 indicates a significant impairment in the patient's quality of life [10]. Most studies of psoriasis investigating induction of remission of the disease take as the primary efficacy variable a 75% improvement in the PASI score from baseline at 3 months. This is often referred to as PASI 75. The fact that most studies use these scoring systems and assess response at 3 months indicates that, at least to some extent, results can be extrapolated across studies. This becomes important when it is recognized that there are very few head-to-head studies that allow direct comparison between therapeutic interventions.

Important differences between psoriasis and rheumatoid arthritis

There is considerable overlap between the systemic drugs used in the treatment of psoriasis and those used for treatment of rheumatoid arthritis (RA). Further, this has been brought into sharp focus by the advent of biologics in which the use of TNFα-blockers has led to a paradigm shift in our ability to treat these two debilitating diseases. Dermatologists are fortunate that much of the toxicity of these drugs has been elucidated prior to their use in psoriasis management. However, it is important to note that there are differences between the two diseases, which indicate that efficacy, tolerability, and safety data cannot be directly extrapolated between the diseases. Amongst the important differences between systemic management of psoriasis and RA are:

- Therapeutic interventions aimed at inhibiting T-cell activity are more successful in the management of psoriasis than in RA. Interestingly, these approaches are rarely of benefit in psoriatic arthritis.
- Many psoriasis patients receiving biological treatments will have received ultraviolet (UV) radiation treatments, including UVB and PUVA (p/soralen plus UVA light), treatments not used in rheumatology. The risk of skin cancer in patients treated with biologics is therefore a matter that requires vigilance and cannot be predicted from previous studies.
- Patients with psoriasis tend to be more obese and to have higher alcohol consumption than those with RA. This has implications for drug metabolism and hepatotoxicity. Interestingly, many dermatologists have reported higher incidences of hepatotoxicity in patients with psoriasis treated with methotrexate than in those with RA.
- The skin is often referred to as the largest organ in the body. When psoriasis is severe, the degree of general inflammation to the patient is great. The implications for drug dosing may therefore be different.

There is a general perception that psoriasis is not a harmful disease and that RA is much more so. Therapeutic interventions, therefore, have to be deemed very safe before given to patients with psoriasis.

Biological therapy for psoriasis

In the USA, four biologics are presently licensed for the treatment of moderate to severe psoriasis: alefacept, efalizumab, etanercept, and infliximab. In Europe, the situation is the same except that alefacept is not licensed. It is anticipated that in the near future adalimumab will also be licensed in the

USA and Europe. These drugs can be broadly subdivided into two groups: (1) those that specifically target T-cell activity (alefacept and efalizumab) and (2) those that target TNFα (etanercept, infliximab, and adalimumab). Importantly, alefacept and efalizumab do not presently have any licensed indications in the fields of rheumatology and gastroenterology. Both of these drugs were developed primarily for the treatment of moderate to severe psoriasis.

References

1 Smith CH and Barker JN. Psoriasis and its management. *BMJ* 2006; **333**: 380–4.
2 Mrowietz U, Elder JT, and Barker JNWN. The importance of disease associations and concomitant therapy for the long term management of psoriasis patients. *Arch Dermatol Res* 2006; **298**: 309–19.
3 Finlay AY and Coles EC. The effect of severe psoriasis on the quality of life of 369 patients. *Br J Dermatol* 1995; **132**: 236–44.
4 Griffiths CME, Camp RDR, and Barker JNWN. Psoriasis. In: Burns T, Breathnach S, Cox N, and Griffiths C (eds) *Rook's Textbook of Dermatology*, 7th edn, pp 1–35. Oxford: Blackwell, 2005.
5 Gelfand JM, Neimann AL, Shin DB, Wang X, Margolis DJ, and Troxel AB. Risk of myocardial infarction in patients with psoriasis. *JAMA* 2006; **296**: 1735–41.
6 Capon F, Munro M, Trembath R, and Barker J. Searching for the MHC psoriasis susceptibility gene. *J Invest Dermatol* 2002; **118**: 745–51.
7 Cargill M, Schrodi SJ, Chang M, *et al*. A large-scale genetic association study confirms *IL12B* and leads to the identification of *IL23R* as psoriasis-risk genes. *Am J Hum Genet* 2007; **80**: 273–90.
8 Capon F, Di Meglio P, Szaub J, *et al*. Sequence variants in the genes for the interleukin-23 receptor (*IL23R*) and its ligand (*IL12B*) confer protection against psoriasis. *Hum Genet* 2007; **122**: 201–6.
9 Griffiths CEM and Barker JNWN. Psoriasis: background and clinical features. *Lancet* 2007; **370**: 263–71.
10 Finlay AY. Current severe psoriasis and the rule of tens. *Br J Dermatol* 2005; **152**: 861–7.

Etanercept (Enbrel)

Chemical properties	Recombinant human TNF receptor p75 Fc fusion protein. There are two receptors for TNF, a 55-kDa protein, TNFR1 (p55), and a 75-kDa protein, TNFR2 (p75), which bind TNF (TNFα) and also lymphotoxin (TNFβ)
Manufacture	Produced in Chinese Hamster Ovary (CHO) cells
Stability	Stable for at least 36 months if stored in the dark at 2–8°C
Pharmacokinetics	After a single 25-mg subcutaneous injection, maximum peak serum concentration (C_{max}) was 1.1 ± 0.6 µg/ml, time to C_{max} 69 ± 34 hours. Mean (SD) half-life was 102(30) hours. After 6 months of 25 mg twice weekly in the same patients ($n=23$), C_{max} was 2.4 ± 1.0 µg/ml, with a 2–7-fold increase in peak serum concentrations. The area under the curve 0–72 hours rose about 4-fold (range 1–17) with repeated dosing. Age and sex had no effect on pharmacokinetics. The effect of renal or hepatic impairment is unknown
Metabolism	Unclear, but thought to be catabolized in a similar manner to normal human immunoglobulin
Drug interactions	There is no information about interactions with methotrexate

Clinical trial data – psoriasis

Study 1 – USA, Phase II (Leonardi et al.) [1] This study was the first large-scale study to confirm the clinical efficacy of etanercept in chronic plaque psoriasis. The critical data concern PASI 75 at 12 weeks. Depending on the dose used, up to approximately 50% of patients achieved PASI 75 at 12 weeks. Importantly, in patients who continued to receive the medication to 24 weeks there was a slight increase in PASI 75 at 24 weeks (59% at the highest dose), indicating that in responders at 12 weeks an increasing benefit over 24 weeks may be anticipated.

Randomized, placebo-controlled, double-blind, dose-finding study; patients with chronic plaque psoriasis, PASI >10, body surface area (BSA) >10%. 652

patients, 67% male, mean age 45.1 years, mean duration of disease 18.7 years, mean baseline PASI 18.4, mean baseline BSA 28.7%.

Treatment	PASI at week 12			PASI at week 24		
	50	75	90	50	75	90
25 mg/week	41%	14%	3%	58%	25%	6%
25 mg twice weekly	58%	34%	12%	70%	44%	20%
50 mg twice weekly	74%	49%	22%	77%	59%	30%
Placebo	14%	4%	1%			

$P < 0.001$ vs placebo at 12 weeks.

Study 2 – USA and Canada, Phase III [2] This phase III study looked at a single high dose (50 mg twice weekly) of etanercept versus placebo over a 12 week period. The results obtained for PASI were essentially identical to those seen in study 1. As well as demonstrating efficacy of this drug and improving psoriasis, the key aspect of this study was that the design included observation of outcomes relating to fatigue and symptoms of depression. The study demonstrated that etanercept, at least at the higher dose, had a significant and clinically meaningful improvement in patient fatigue and in symptoms of depression. 34% of the patients also have psoriatic arthritis.

Randomized, placebo-controlled, double-blind fixed-dose study, chronic plaque psoriasis, PASI > 10. 618 patients, 68% male, mean age 45.7 years, mean duration of disease 20 years, mean baseline PASI 18.2.

Treatment	PASI at week 12		
	50	75	90
50 mg twice weekly	74%	47%	21%
Placebo	14%	5%	1%

Study 3 – USA, Canada, Europe, Phase III [3] This phase III study was the first to report data outside the USA and Canada. Europe was a major recruitment site. The 12-week data in this study are consistent with those in studies 1 and 2. A key element, however, was the extension study between 12 and 24 weeks, when all patients received etanercept 25 mg twice weekly. Importantly, the data demonstrate that clinical benefit is maintained in those individuals who received 50 mg twice weekly for 12 weeks. These data support the dosing used in the label, namely for the first 12 weeks patients should receive 50 mg twice weekly and 25 mg twice weekly subsequently for up to 24 weeks.

Another important facet of this study is the fact that 89% of the patients had previously received treatment with either systemic therapy or phototherapy for their disease. In other words, they had previously been exposed to other systemic therapies; however, this did not have any adverse influence on efficacy outcome. This is consistent with the clinical use of the drug in patients in whom systemic therapies have failed for one reason or another.

Randomized, placebo-controlled, multicentre, double-blind study, BSA >10%, PASI >10. 583 patients, 66% male, median age 45 years, median duration of psoriasis 19 years, median BSA 23%, median PASI 16.4.

Treatment	PASI at week 12			PASI at week 24		
	50	75	90	50	75	90
25 mg twice weekly	64%	34%	11%		42%	
50 mg twice weekly	77%	49%	21		50%	
Placebo	9%	3%	1%		26%	

Infliximab (Remicade)

Administration	Intravenous infusion in normal saline (sodium chloride 0.9%) over 2 hours
Chemical properties	Recombinant human–murine chimaeric IgG1 monoclonal antibody
Manufacture	Produced in cell line by continuous perfusion
Stability	Stable for at least 36 months if stored in the dark at 2–8°C
Pharmacokinetics	Single dosing of 3–10 mg/kg in RA and 5 mg/kg in Crohn's disease indicate median terminal half-life of 8–9.5 days. Single 3–20-mg/kg intravenous dosing shows linear dose–blood level relationship, indicating mainly intravascular compartment distribution. Eight weeks after a dose given during regular therapy, stable blood levels of approximately 0.5–6 µg/ml were seen, with no systemic accumulation of drug. The development of anti-infliximab antibodies substantially increased clearance
Metabolism	Unclear, but thought to be catabolized in a similar manner to normal human immunoglobulin
Drug interactions	Methotrexate and other immunosuppressant medications probably decrease the formation of antibodies against infliximab and increase plasma concentrations of infliximab

Clinical trial data – psoriasis

Study 1 – USA, Phase II [4] Randomized, placebo-controlled, double-blind, single-centre study. BSA >5%, no minimum PASI, but disease described as moderate to severe. 33 patients, 67% male, mean age 43 years, PASI 23.

Treatment	Week 10 PASI 75	PGA
5 mg/kg*	82%	82%
10 mg/kg*	73%	91%
Placebo*	18%	18%

*By intravenous infusion at weeks 0, 2, and 6. PGA, physician global assessment.

Although this was a small, early, phase II study, it was pivotal in the development of anti-TNFα therapy for psoriasis. The only previously recorded use of anti-TNFα treatment for psoriasis was an isolated case report from the same group. In contrast to most other studies, the primary efficacy variable used here was a dynamic physcan global assessment (PGA). However, the PASI scores were also recorded, from which a PASI 75 was derived. This study also reported the data at 10 weeks, which, although different most other studies (data at 12 weeks), allows for reasonable comparison. Study 2 (see below) was a direct consequence of study 1. The key observation in this study was the dramatically effective nature of infliximab, at least in the short term.

Note: Infliximab was given by intravenous infusion, unlike the other TNFα therapies for psoriasis.

Study 2 – USA, Phase II/III [5] Randomized, double-blind, placebo-controlled, multicentre trial, BSA >10%, PASI >12. 249 patients, 68% male, mean age 45 years, mean duration of psoriasis 17 years, mean BSA 27%, mean PASI 19.

Treatment	PASI at week 10		
	50	75	90
Infliximab*			
3 mg/kg	83%	72%	45%
5 mg/kg	97%	88%	57%
Placebo*	22%	6%	2%

*By intravenous infusion at weeks 0, 2, and 6.

Study 2 is the pivotal study of infliximab for psoriasis. The efficacy data are similar to those obtained in study 1. It is of note that essentially all patients received moderate benefit (PASI >50% improvement), at least in the short term (10 weeks).

This study also revealed that three infusions of infliximab at weeks 0, 2, and 6 can provide benefit over many weeks without redosing. Intermittent dosing versus continuous dosing remains the subject of investigation.

Study 3 – Canada and Europe, Phase III [6] Multicentre, randomized, placebo-controlled, double-blind study, with crossover arm. BSA >10%, PASI >12. 378 patients, 61% male, mean age 43 years, mean duration of psoriasis 18.7 years, mean BSA 34%, mean PASI 23.

Treatment	PASI at week 10			PASI at week 24			PASI at week 50		
	50	75	90	50	75	90	50	75	90
Infliximab 50 mg/kg*	91%	80%	57%	90%	82%	58%			
Placebo*	8%	3%	1%	6%	4%	1%	90†	77†	50†

*By infusion at weeks 0, 2, 6, and then every 8 weeks.
†Crossover to infliximab at week 24.

The above study represents key data in establishing the role of infliximab in the management of chronic plaque psoriasis as a maintenance therapy. The data demonstrate that at 5 mg/kg (licensed dosage), short-term data as revealed in studies 1 and 2 are replicated. The critical new data presented in study 3 are long term (to 50 weeks), and demonstrate that at week 24 the effect is maintained. At week 50, although the majority of patients continued to do well on the drug, there was some loss of effect, at least in some patients. Also determined by study 3 is the fact that infliximab appears to be an excellent treatment for psoriatic male dystrophy. From the safety point of view, the long-term data identified in this study revealed no new safety concerns for infliximab in the psoriatic population.

Study 4 – USA and Canada, Phase III/IV [7] Multicentre, randomized study comparing treatment every 8 weeks with 'as needed' treatment over 50 weeks; BSA >10%, PASI >12. 835 patients, 66% male, mean age 44 years, mean duration of psoriasis 18 years, mean BSA 28%, mean PASI 20.

Treatment	PASI at week 10		PASI at week 50	
	75	50	75	90
Infliximab				
3 mg/kg continuous*	70%	55%	44%	25%
3 mg/kg on demand†	–	60%	25%	9%
5 mg/kg continuous*	75%	72%	54%	34%
5 mg/kg on demand†		73%	38%	10%
Placebo	2%			

*Infusions at weeks 0, 2, 6, and every 8 weeks thereafter.
†Infusions at weeks 0, 2, 6, and then as per protocol (see text).

Study 4 represents an attempt to compare intermittent but continuous dosing of infliximab (infusion every 2 months) with dosing dependent upon clinical lead. To achieve this, clinical need has to be defined as a PASI improvement of less than 75% compared with baseline. This was assessed monthly and, when inadequate clinical improvement was noted, the patient was infused with infliximab. The study clearly demonstrates the continuous intermittent infusions represent a more optimal way of managing moderate to severe psoriasis. A secondary outcome of this study confirms the findings of previous studies, namely that 5 mg/kg is better than 3 mg/kg. With respect to this parameter, the new observation here is that 5 mg/kg is better at week 50 as well as at week 10. The licence for infliximab is for continuous intermittent dosing. This study is the only randomized, placebo-controlled trial of adalimumab in the treatment of psoriasis so far reported. However, the study clearly demonstrates the efficacy of adalimumab. Significant benefit is obtained by week 12 and this effect is maintained for at least 60 weeks. The study further demonstrates that, although 40 mg weekly by subcutaneous injection of adalimumab works more rapidly than 40 mg every other week, the difference in effect with respect to maintenance treatment (to 60 weeks) is very small. The European Medicines Evaluation Agency (EMEA) licence for adalimumab for the treatment of moderate to severe psoriasis uses alternate-week dosing.

Adalimumab (Humira)

Chemical properties	Recombinant human IgG1 monoclonal antibody, 148 kDa
Manufacture	Produced in Chinese Hamster Ovary cells
Stability	Stable for at least 24 months if stored in the dark at 2–8°C
Pharmacokinetics	After a single 40-mg subcutaneous injection, average peak serum concentration was 4.7 µg/ml after 5.4 days. Average bioavailability compared with intravenous dosing is 64%. Half-life is between 10 and 20 days. The clearance in patients with moderate to severe psoriasis is probably lower than in RA studies
Metabolism	Unclear, but thought to be catabolized in a similar manner to normal human immunoglobulin. In patients receiving adalimumab monotherapy, clearance in patients with RA is faster than in those with moderate to severe psoriasis
Drug interactions	Methotrexate probably decreases the clearance rate of adalimumab, although this does not depend on the dose of methotrexate (tested range 5–30 mg). Adalimumab does not alter methotrexate concentrations

Clinical trial data – psoriasis

Study 1 – USA and Canada, Phase II [8] Multicentre, randomized, double-blind, placebo-controlled study, with extension arm; BSA >5%. 147 patients, 67% male, mean age 44.5 years, mean duration of psoriasis 19 years, mean BSA 27%, mean PASI 15.5.

Treatment	PASI 75 Week 12	Week 24	Week 36	Week 60
Adalimumab				
40 mg e.o.w.	53%	64%	62%	56%
40 mg weekly	80%	72%	65%	64%
Placebo	4%			

e.o.w., every other week.

Study 2 – USA and Canada, Phase III [9] Multicentre, randomized, double-blind, placebo-controlled study, with 2 : 1 randomization to adalimumab 80 mg week, then 40 mg every other week (e.o.w.) or placebo injections until week 16. PASI 75 responders from either group then received open-label adalimumab 40 mg e.o.w. until week 33, when PASI 75 responders who had received adalimumab from week 0 were re-randomized to receive adalimumab 40 mg e.o.w. or placebo injection until week 52, i.e. a blinded treatment withdrawal arm. At week 16 the patients from either placebo or active therapy groups who did not achieve a PASI 75 response were enrolled in a separate open-label extension study.

BSA > 10%; PASI ±12; PGA at least moderate
n = 1212 Male = 66% Mean age = 45 years
Mean duration of psoriasis = 18 years
Mean BSA = 26% Mean PASI = 19

	PASI and PGA (% patients clear or minimal)								
	Week 12			Week 16			Week 24		
	PGA	75	90	PGA	75	90	PGA	75	90
Placebo	4%	5%	2%	-	7%	2%	N/A	N/A	N/A
Adalimumab	60%	68%	37%	60%	73%	45%	60%	77%	49%

P <0.001 adalimumab vs placebo at 12 and 16 weeks.

Safety. A numerical increase in non-malignant skin tumours in the adalimumab group up to week 16 (4) vs placebo (1). No other new adverse events compared with those known from other indications.

Study 3 – Europe and Canada, Phase III [10] Phase III randomized, double-blind, double-dummy, placebo-controlled study comparing adalimumab subcutaneous injections with oral methotrexate and placebo in patient with moderate to severe psoriasis in a 2 : 2: 1 ratio to adalimumab, methotrexate, or placebo, for 16 weeks. Adalimumab 80 mg at week 0, then 40 mg e.o.w. Oral methotrexate as a single weekly dose initiated at 7.5 mg per week at week 0, increased to 10 mg per week at week 2, and increased to 15 mg per week at week 4 for all patients. At week 8 onward, patients who achieved at least a 50% reduction in Psoriasis Area and Severity Index (PASI 50) response maintained their current dosages (15 mg per week maximum) for the duration of the study. At week 8, patients who did not achieve a PASI 50 response had methotrexate dosage increased to 20 mg per week. At week 12, patients not achieving a PASI 50 response and who had a < PASI 50 responses at week 8 had further dosage increase to 25 mg per week for the duration of the study. Patients who achieved ≥12 PASI 50 responses at week 12 maintained their current dosages (20 mg per week maximum) for the duration of the study. Oral medication dosages were also adjusted to alanine aminotransferase, aspartate aminotransferase, serum creatinine, and blood cell count between week 2 and week 15, if necessary, and could be withheld or reduced at any time, as deemed appropriate by the safety assessors.

BSA ≥ 10% PASI ≥10
$n = 271$ Male = 66%   Mean age = 41.5 years
Mean duration of psoriasis = 18.5 years
Mean BSA = 32.1%   Mean PASI = 19.7

	PASI and PGA (% patients clear or minimal)						
	Week 4		Week 12		Week 16		
	PGA	Mean % change	PGA	Mean % change PASI	PGA	75	100	Mean % change PASI
Placebo	2%	15%	9.4%	21%	11%	19%	2%	21%
MTX	4%	22%	21%	49%	30%	36%	7%	54%
ADA	16%†	56%*	67%*	81%*	73%*	79%*	17%‡	81%*

*P <0.001 adalimumab vs placebo at 4,12 and 16 weeks.
†P = 0.007 adalimumab vs placebo.
‡P = 0.004 vs placebo.

The mean ± SD weekly dosages of oral medication in the methotrexate group were 14.2 ± 3.0 mg at week 4, 16.8 ± 3.0 mg at week 8, 18.8 ± 4.8 mg at week 12, and 19.2 ± 4.9 mg at week 15. Eighty-nine of 95 (94%) patients in the methotrexate group received a methotrexate dosage of ≥15 mg at week 12. Six patients (6%) received a dosage of <15 mg at week 12 because of elevations of alanine aminotransferase or aspartate aminotransferase concentrations >1.5 times the upper limit of normal value, which necessitated decreasing the methotrexate dosage. Treatment compliance (mean ± SD) was high for use of both oral (99.7 ± 2.5%) and injectable (97.2 ± 8.7%) study medications.

Efalizumab (Raptiva)

Chemical properties	Efalizumab is a recombinant humanized monoclonal (IgG1 kappa) antibody
Manufacture	Produced in Chinese Hamster Ovary cells
Stability	Stable for at least 3 years if refrigerated and protected from light. After reconstitution with solvent, immediate use is recommended
Pharmacokinetics	The drug is provided in a powder form. Following subcutaneous administration, peak plasma concentrations are reached after 1–2 days. At the recommended dose (see below) steady state is observed at week 4. Elimination half-life is between 5 and 10 days
Drug interactions	There are no consistent drug interactions reported with efalizumab. However, early data on the effects of vaccination in patients receiving efalizumab indicate that the immune response to vaccines may be reduced. It is therefore recommended that treatment with efalizumab should be withheld for 8 weeks prior to patients receiving live vaccines. The drug should not be introduced for at least 2 weeks after vaccination
Mechanism	Efalizumab binds specifically to the CD11a subunit of lymphocyte functional associated antigen 1 (LFA-1) on the surface of T cells, thereby inhibiting their binding to intercellular adhesion molecule 1 (ICAM-1). By this mechanism it inhibits trafficking of T cells to sites of inflammation (through the binding of T cells to endothelial cells), and by inhibiting T-cell antigen presentation by preventing binding to antigen-presenting cells. Pharmacodynamic studies validate these proposed mechanism of action by, for example, revealing absolute increases in counts of circulating leucocytes after efalizumab treatment

Clinical trial data – psoriasis

Efalizumab is recommended for the 'treatment of adult patients with moderate to severe chronic plaque psoriasis who have failed to respond to, or who have a contraindication to, or are intolerant to other systemic therapies including ciclosporin, methotrexate and PUVA'. The above is the European indication. It is different in the USA, where the licensed indication is 'for the treatment of adult patients with chronic moderate to severe plaque psoriasis who are candidates for systemic therapy or phototherapy'. The key difference is that, in Europe, patients will be expected to have received other systemic therapies prior to receiving efalizumab therapy. The same holds for the other biologics as well. The drug is given by subcutaneous injection once weekly. In week 1, the dose is 0.7 mg/kg bodyweight, followed by weekly subcutaneous injections of 1 mg/kg bodyweight.

Five clinical studies of efalizumab have been reported in moderate to severe psoriasis. These indicate that 30% of patients can expect to achieve 75% improvement in PASI by week 12. Evidence exists from longer-term studies that, in patients achieving a PASI 50 at week 12, further improvement may occur to week 24. It is recommended that the drug is not used beyond 12 weeks if a reduction in PASI of 50 has not been achieved. It appears that exacerbation of psoriasis is more common in this subset.

Study 1 – USA and Canada, Phase III [11] Multicentre, placebo-controlled, double-blind study, PASI >12, BSA >10%. 597 patients, 65% male, mean age 46 years, mean duration of disease 19 years, mean baseline PASI 20.

Treatment	PASI at week 12			PASI at week 24		
	50	75	90	50	75	90
Efalizumab						
1 mg/kg	52%	22%	4%	95%	78%	32%
2 mg/kg	57%	28%	6%	90%	77%	31%
Placebo	16%	5%	<1%	40%	20%	2%

This study represented the pivotal phase III study for efalizumab. As for the etanercept studies, the key factor is the PASI 75 at week 12; both doses of efalizumab were more effective than placebo. The week 24 data refer only to patients who had achieved a PASI 75 at week 12. In other words, the study examined maintenance of remission. It is clear from these data, firstly that effect was lost in patients who were maintained on placebo at weeks 12 and 24, but that effect was maintained in those who continued to receive efalizumab – at least in the majority of patients. Finally, there was no difference in efficacy between 1 mg/kg efalizumab weekly and 2 mg/kg efalizumab weekly. On the basis of this evidence, 1 mg/kg weekly efalizumab is used as the standard dose.

Study 2 – USA and Canada, Phase III [12] Multicentre, randomized, double-blind, placebo-controlled study; PASI >12, BSA >10%. 556 patients, 69% male, mean age 45 years, mean baseline PASI 19, BSA 2.8%, mean duration of disease 19 years.

Treatment	PASI at week 12	
	50	75
Efalizumab 1 mg/kg per week	59%	27%
Placebo	14%	4%

This study reported 12-week data of efalizumab at a dose of 1 mg/kg per week. The results were essentially identical to those found in study 1.

Study 3 – USA and Canada, Phase III [13] Multicentre, randomized, placebo-controlled, double-blind study; PASI >12, BSA >10%. 498 patients, 72& male. mean age 44 years, mean PASI at baseline 19, BSA 29%, mean duration of disease 18 years.

Treatment	PASI at week 12			PASI at week 24		
	50	75	90	50	75	90
Efalizumab						
1 mg/kg	61.1%	38.9%	12.3%	45.6%	21.1%	8.8%
2 mg/kg	51.2%	26.5%	4.8%	53.0%	19.7%	0%
Placebo	14.7%	2.4%	1.2%	23.3%	6.7%	1.7%

This study again confirms clinical benefit of efalizumab in patients treated for up to 12 weeks. The data presented for week 24 refer to patients who failed to achieve a PASI 75 despite being on active drug up to week 12. The key information here is that 20% of patients achieved a PASI 75 over and above the number achieving it at week 12. This indicates that continuing the drug for 24 weeks provides additional clinical benefit over that observed at 12 weeks. This study was performed in a number of countries outside the USA and Canada. The data are consistent with those found in studies 1–3.

The important message derived from this paper is that the study included a separate analysis of patients described as 'high need'. This was defined as 'unsuitability of at least two systemic treatments due to lack of efficacy, intolerance or contraindication'. A separate analysis of this large subgroup within the study population produced similar findings to those from the total group. This indicates that efalizumab is effective in patients for whom standard therapies cannot be used. As such, this study provides data supporting its labelled use in Europe.

Study 4 – Canada, Europe, Australia, Israel, Phase III [14] Multinational, randomized, doubled-blind, placebo-controlled study; PASI >12, BSA >10%. 793 patients, 67% male, mean age 45 years, mean PASI at baseline 24, BSA 37%, mean duration of disease 21 years.

Treatment	PASI response week 12 Total group		'High need' group	
	50	75	50	75
Efalizumab 1 mg/kg	59.7%	31.4%	52.0%	29.5%
Placebo	14.4%	4.2%	12.0%	2.7%

Safety of efalizumab

Pre-treatment it is recommended so that severe systemic and local infections are excluded. Reliable contraception is advised, although there are no adequate data regarding the use of efalizumab in pregnant women to assess the risk accurately. However, it is known that immunoglobulins can cross the placental barrier and be excreted in human milk. Breastfeeding mothers should therefore also be excluded from efalizumab therapy. Given the possibility of haematological and hepatic biochemical changes with efalizumab therapy, baseline laboratory data should be collected.

Flu-like symptoms, including headache, fever, chills, nausea, and myalgia, may be observed during efalizumab treatment. These tend to occur in the first 2 or 3 weeks after treatment has been initiated and probably represent a form of cytokine release. This explains the lower dose in week 1.

Occasionally mild changes in liver function test results (particularly alanine transaminase) are seen, but rarely require action. Thrombocytopenia has been reported uncommonly and may occur early or late in disease management. Importantly, no increased rate of neoplasia or tuberculosis has been seen in efalizumab-treated patients. Postmarketing surveillance has identified rare cases of an inflammatory polyradiculoneuropathy occurring in patients receiving efalizumab. When these events occur, the drug should be ceased immediately and appropriate measures taken. Finally, cases of inflammatory arthritis have been observed during treatment or after discontinuation of efalizumab. Further information is required to assess the relevance of the drug to the onset of these symptoms.

During treatment it is essential that patients are monitored for signs of infection and asked about the onset of any adverse events. Efficacy in the form of a formal PASI assessment should be performed at 12 weeks, and only if a PASI 50 is achieved should the drug be continued. After treatment, when the drug is discontinued, close follow-up should be undertaken to exclude relapse or rebound. It is recommended that the drug is not used beyond 12 weeks if a reduction in PASI of 50 has not been achieved. It appears that exacerbation of psoriasis is more common in this subset. In this instance, the introduction of an alternative suitable psoriasis treatment is recommended. Patients should be made aware of these potential adverse events.

Alefacept (Amevive)

This drug is not available in the EU.

Chemical properties	Alefacept is a dimeric fusion protein consisting of the extracellular CD2 binding portion of human leucocyte functional antigen 3 (LFA-3) linked to the Fc portion of human IgG1
Manufacture	Produced in Chinese Hamster Ovary cells
Stability	Stable for at least 36 months if stored in the dark at 2–8°C
Pharmacokinetics	The drug is provided in powder form. The mean elimination half-life is approximately 10–15 days in adults. It is administered after reconstitution of 15 mg lyophilized powder, reconstituted in 0.6 ml supplied diluant (sterile water for injection). The drug is given weekly for 12 weeks, administered by intramuscular injection. The pharmacokinetics of alefacept have not been studied in the paediatric population
Metabolism	
Drug interactions	There are no consistent drug interactions reported with alefacept
Mechanism	Alefacept interferes with lymphocyte activation by binding specifically to the lymphocyte antigen CD2 and thereby inhibiting LFA-3–CD2 interactions. The majority of T lymphocytes and psoriatic lesions are of the memory effector phenotype, and the consequences of LFA-3–CD2 interference is lack of activation of these cells, which are thought to be important in pathophysiology with consequent inhibition of release of inflammatory cytokines such as interferon-γ. Alefacept also leads to a reduction in CD2-positive T-cell subsets, which include both CD45 RO-positive memory cells and natural killer cells

Clinical trial data – psoriasis

Alefacept is recommended for the treatment of adult patients with moderate to severe chronic plaque psoriasis who are candidates for systemic therapy or phototherapy. As stated above, the drug is not available within the EU.

Two randomized, double-blind, placebo-controlled studies in adults with chronic plaque psoriasis have been performed. These studies indicate that between 14% and 21% of patients achieved a 75% reduction in PASI 2 weeks after a 12-week course of treatment, and approximately 40% achieved a 50% reduction in PASI. Patients receiving a second 12-week course of alefacept (15 mg weekly by intramuscular injection) had an increased response.

Alefacept induces dose-dependent reductions in circulating lymphocyte counts. Hence it is recommended that CD4+ T-lymphocyte counts should be monitored every 2 weeks during the 12-week treatment period and used to guide dosing. Importantly, patients should have a normal CD4+ T-lymphocyte count prior to initial or subsequent courses of treatment with alefacept. If CD4+ lymphocyte counts are below 250 cells/µl, alefacept dosing should be withheld and weekly monitoring instituted. Alefacept should be discontinued if the CD4+ T-lymphocyte count remains below 250 cells/µl for 1 month.

Because of the immunosuppressive effects of alefacept, the drug should not be administered to patients with a clinically important infection. Patients should be monitored for signs and symptoms of infection during the course of treatment. Alefacept should not be administered to patients infected with HIV. The drug may reduce CD4+ T-cell counts, and may accelerate to disease progression or increase the complications of disease in these patients.

Alefacept should not be administered to patients with a history of systemic malignancy and should be used with caution in patients with a high risk of malignancy. If a patient develops a malignancy, alefacept should be discontinued.

The safety and efficacy of vaccines, specifically live or live-attenuated vaccines, administered to patients being treated with alefacept has not been studied. A small study of patients with chronic plaque psoriasis indicated that the ability to mount an immune response to tetanus toxide (recall antigen) and an experimental neoantigen was preserved in the patients undergoing alefacept treatment.

With respect to pregnancy, the US Food and Drug Administration advises that, because the risk to the fetal immune system and postnatal immune function in humans is unknown, alefacept should be used during pregnancy only if clearly needed. If pregnancy occurs while taking alefacept, continued use of the drug should be assessed. It is not known whether alefacept is excreted in human milk. Thus, a decision should be made of whether to discontinue breastfeeding while taking the drug, or whether to discontinue taking the drug, balancing the importance of it to the nursing mother.

Postmarketing experience includes reports of hepatic injury, including an asymptomatic increase in transaminase levels, fatty infiltration of the liver, hepatitis, and decompensation of cirrhosis with liver failure. Although the exact relationship between these and the use of alefacept has not been established, the drug should be discontinued in patients who develop significant clinical signs of hepatic injury.

Some 16% of patients receiving intramuscular alefacept in clinical trials reported injection site reactions. These were generally mild, occurring on single occasions; they can best be dealt with by rotation of the injection sites.

References

1 Leonardi CL, Powers JL, Matheson RT, *et al.*; Etanercept Psoriasis Study Group. Etanercept as monotherapy in patients with psoriasis. *N Engl J Med* 2003; **349**: 2014–22.
2 Tyring S, Gottlieb A, Papp K, *et al.* Etanercept and clinical outcomes, fatigue, and depression in psoriasis: double-blind placebo-controlled randomised phase III trial. *Lancet* 2006; **367**: 29–35.
3 Papp KA, Tyring S, Lahfa M, *et al.*; Etanercept Psoriasis Study Group. A global phase III randomized controlled trial of etanercept in psoriasis: safety, efficacy, and effect of dose reduction. *Br J Dermatol* 2005; **152**: 1304–12.
4 Chaudhari U, Romano P, Mulcahy LD, Dooley LT, Baker DG, and Gottlieb AB. Efficacy and safety of infliximab monotherapy for plaque-type psoriasis: a randomised trial. *Lancet* 2001; **357**: 1842–7.
5 Gottlieb AB, Evans R, Li S, *et al.* Infliximab induction therapy for patients with severe plaque-type psoriasis: a randomized, double-blind, placebo-controlled trial. *J Am Acad Dermatol* 2004; **51**: 534–42.
6 Reich K, Nestle FO, Papp K, *et al.*; EXPRESS Study Investigators. Infliximab induction and maintenance therapy for moderate-to-severe psoriasis: a phase III, multicentre, double-blind trial. *Lancet* 2005; **366**: 1367–74.
7 Menter A, Feldman SR, Weinstein GD, *et al.* A randomized comparison of continuous vs. intermittent infliximab maintenance regimens over 1 year in the treatment of moderate-to-severe plaque psoriasis. *J Am Acad Dermatol* 2007; **56**: 31.e1–15.
8 Gordon KB, Langley RG, Leonardi C, *et al.* Clinical response to adalimumab treatment in patients with moderate to severe psoriasis: double-blind, randomized controlled trial and open-label extension study. *J Am Acad Dermatol* 2006; **55**: 598–606.
9 Menter A, Tyring SK, Gordon K, *et al.* Adalimumab therapy for moderate to severe psoriasis: a randomized, controlled phase III trial. *J Am Acad Dermatol* 2008; **58**: 106–15. Epub 2007 Oct 23.
10 Saurat JH, Stingl G, Dubertret L, *et al.* Efficacy and safety results from the randomized controlled comparative study of adalimumab vs. methotrexate vs. placebo in patients with psoriasis (CHAMPION). *Br J Dermatol.* 2008; **158**: 558–66. Epub 2007 Nov 28.

11 Lebwohl M, Tyring SK, Hamilton TK, *et al.*; Efalizumab Study Group. A novel targeted T-cell modulator, efalizumab, for plaque psoriasis. *N Engl J Med* 2003; **349**: 2004–13.
12 Gordon KB, Papp KA, **Hamilton TK,** *et al.*; Efalizumab Study Group. Efalizumab for patients with moderate to severe plaque psoriasis: a randomized controlled trial. *JAMA* 2003; **290**: 3073–80.
13 Leonardi CL, Papp KA, Gordon KB, *et al.*; Efalizumab Study Group. Extended efalizumab therapy improves chronic plaque psoriasis: results from a randomized phase III trial. *J Am Acad Dermatol* 2005; **52**: 425–33.
14 Dubertret L, Sterry W, Bos JD, *et al.*; CLEAR Multinational Study Group. CLinical Experience Acquired with the efalizumab (Raptiva) (CLEAR) trial in patients with moderate-to-severe plaque psoriasis: results from a phase III international randomized, placebo-controlled trial. *Br J Dermatol* 2006; **155**: 170–81.

4
Gastroenterology

Biological therapy in inflammatory bowel disease and Crohn's disease

Chronic inflammatory bowel diseases (IBD), Crohn's disease (CD), and ulcerative colitis (UC) affect more than one million Americans. The symptoms of CD can range from mild to severe, with a burden that can be bothersome to disabling. This disease results in inflammation of the ileum (the most distal part of the small intestine) and the colon, and can cause nutritional deficiencies, intestinal blockage, fistulas, and scarring, and result in the need for surgical procedures to correct complications, such as blockage or abscesses. In patients with severe CD, surgical resection is necessary. Illustrating the progressive nature of CD, over 20 years the cumulative probability of surgical intervention in CD is greater than 80%. Once surgery is necessary in an individual patient, the probability of a second and third operation becomes increasingly greater [1].

For patients with CD who present with active signs and symptoms, the immediate therapeutic goal is to induce clinical remission as quickly as possible. However, once remission is induced, subsequent flares are the rule unless maintenance therapy is initiated and continued. This requires both effective induction and maintenance therapies that have appropriate risk–benefit profiles. Treatment efficacy of these therapies is measured through the Crohn's Disease Activity Index (CDAI), which is a composite score of clinical symptoms (e.g. diarrhoea, abdominal pain) and signs (e.g. abdominal mass, extraintestinal sites of inflammation, weight loss, and anaemia) that has been well validated in numerous clinical trials of therapeutic interventions in CD.

Inflammation in UC begins in the distal rectum, is uniform and continuous, with no intervening areas of normal mucosa. Clinically, patients with UC suffer from diarrhoea, rectal bleeding, weight loss, and fever. Following a first attack of UC, more than 70% of patients will experience relapses that follow a chronic intermittent or chronic continuous course. Patients with UC have an increased risk of carcinoma when compared with the risk in the general population. The pharmacological management of UC is aimed at reducing colonic inflammation and controlling symptoms; and consists mainly of anti-inflammatory and immunosuppressive therapies. When pharmacological management is not effective, proctocolectomy is the only alternative. Although advances in surgical therapy have provided more satisfactory outcomes for patients with UC, colectomy is associated with a variety of surgical complications (including abscess, anastomotic leaks, obstruction, chronic pouchitis, sexual dysfunction, female infertility, and poor functional results) that can result in repeated surgery, diminished quality of life, and death. Ultimately, colectomy is necessary in 25–40% of patients over the course of disease.

IBD pathogenesis in a clinical context

Recent advances in understanding the pathogenesis of CD and UC have underpinned the development of new biological therapies. We will briefly review advances in the understanding of pathophysiology of IBD that forms the rationale for new biological therapies. A simplistic paradigm for IBD pathogenesis is that, in a genetically predisposed host, varied stimuli from the external environment trigger an overactive mucosal immune response, leading to chronic inflammatory changes in the intestine. Of the environmental factors that initiate and perpetuate mucosal inflammation in IBD, the one that has attracted the most recent attention is the role of the normal enteric microbial flora. The normal intestine is colonized with 10 to 100 microbes for every mammalian cell in the human body. The microbial flora is separated by a single layer of intestinal epithelial cells from the largest immune organ in the body – the mucosal (or intestinal) immune system. In most cases, this enormous and diverse biomass of microbes lives in peace with the mucosal immune system, but in IBD there is inappropriate activation of mucosal immune responses against the enteric microbial flora, initiating and perpetuating inflammation in the gut [2].

Several defined immunological abnormalities have been targeted for therapeutic intervention in human IBD. Intestinal inflammation in IBD is characterized by: (1) secretion of cytokines and other inflammatory products from activated immune cells, which in turn leads to injury of the intestine and abnormal healing response; (2) activation of inflammatory T-cell populations, resulting in perpetuation of the inflammatory state; and (3) increased trafficking to the intestine of inflammatory leucocytes. For example, the cytokine tumour necrosis factor (TNF) is a pivotal inflammatory protein that is overproduced in IBD and contributes to many aspects of the unregulated immune responses in the gut [3]. As will be discussed, antibodies directed against TNF represent the prototypic biological therapy in IBD and other chronic inflammatory disorders.

TNF inhibition: immunological and clinical rationale

Despite longstanding experience with conventional agents in IBD, numerous unmet medical needs remain. The majority of patients will not maintain remission with any conventional agent, and there is no clear evidence that even immunomodulators such as azathioprine, 6-mercaptopurine, or methotrexate fundamentally alter the natural course of the disease. Hence, there remains considerable interest in developing new biological therapies that target inflammatory pathways critical to the pathogenesis of IBD.

The prototypic biological therapies are the anti-TNF agents. TNF is a potent, multifunctional mediator of inflammation and a number of inflammatory diseases including CD, UC, rheumatoid arthritis, psoriasis, psoriatic arthritis, and ankylosing spondylitis. Overproduction of TNF plays an important role in the initiation and maintenance of a cascade of inflammatory events that affect multiple cell and tissue types, which in IBD leads to increased inflammation of the intestinal mucosa and tissue destruction.

Since anti-TNF therapy with infliximab was approved for the treatment of CD, there has been an expanding clinical data set regarding the safety and efficacy of various anti-TNF strategies, including the use of chimaeric (infliximab) and fully human (adalimumab) monoclonal antibodies, and a pegylated Fab fragment (certilizumab pegol).

Assessment of 'top-down' versus 'step-up' strategies in CD

The prevailing therapeutic strategy in CD has been called a 'step-up' approach; that is, treatment progresses from 5-aminosalicylic acid (5-ASA), antibiotics, and topical and/or systemic corticosteroids through immunomodulators, and culminates with anti-TNF therapy. The premise is that conventional agents should be used to treat patients who have mild disease, whereas those who do not respond should be switched to more potent agents, which may be more effective, but necessitate increased need for monitoring, cost, and toxicity concerns. Despite conventional treatment, the course of CD often progresses to the development of complications (fibrosis, stricture, fistula, perforation) and the need for surgery. Accordingly, an alternative strategy, called 'top-down' therapy, has been proposed. In this case, more potent agents are introduced early in the course of the disease to arrest inflammation, promote mucosal healing, and prevent complications that may over the long term result in structural damage and disability.

A randomized controlled study compared top-down therapy with classical step-up therapy in 133 patients with CD with relatively early (<4 years' duration) active disease [4]. Patients were initially randomized to top-down treatment with three infusions of infliximab (weeks 0, 2, and 6) and azathioprine 2–2.5 mg/kg/day, or to step-up treatment with prednisone 40 mg/day. In the top-down group, patients who relapsed were treated with repeat infliximab infusions and then corticosteroids. In the step-up group, azathioprine was added with repeated need for corticosteroids or if the patient developed a dependency on corticosteroids, and infliximab was given only after failure of immunosuppression. Remission (CDAI <150 without steroid use and no bowel resection) was attained in 60% of patients in the top-down group versus 41% of patients in the step-up group at 6 months ($P=0.03$), and in 61% and 50%, respectively, at 12 months ($P=0.19$). At 12 months, 17% of patients in the step-up group were still receiving corticosteroids compared with none in the top-down group ($P<0.001$). The difference between the top-down and step-up groups in immunosuppressant use began to narrow after 60 weeks as patients in the step-up group began receiving azathioprine and infliximab. After 2 years, an endoscopic substudy revealed complete ulcer disappearance in 71% of the patients who received top-down treatment and in 30% of those who received step-up treatment ($P<0.001$) [5]. Therefore, top-down therapy with infliximab was superior to step-up therapy with conventional agents in terms of treatment success at 6 months and corticosteroid sparing throughout the study, and also demonstrated superior mucosal healing at 2 years.

However, given short- and long-term toxicity, cost issues, and the fact that approximately 20% of patients with CD will do well over the long term on conventional therapies, most physicians are not yet ready to commit all such patients to a top-down approach. Therefore, identification of clinical parameters and biomarkers that will predict an aggressive disease course and long-term response to TNF inhibitors is paramount to translate the 'top-down' concept into widespread use in clinical practice.

Future directions/future biologics

Several other agents with varying molecular targets show promise in phase II and III studies. Natalizumab is a recombinant humanized IgG4 monoclonal antibody against α_4 integrin that blocks $\alpha_4\beta_1$ and $\alpha_4\beta_7$, thereby preventing the egress of inflammatory leucocyte populations to sites of inflammation including the gut. Natalizumab has shown promise as an induction, maintenance, and steroid-sparing therapy in phase III trials in CD [6,7].

Originally approved by the US Food and Drug Administration (FDA) in multiple sclerosis (MS), natalizumab was temporarily withdrawn from the market following three reports of fatal progressive multifocal leucoencephalopathy (PML) in two patients with MS who were also receiving interferon-β and in onw patient with CD and prior exposure to azathioprine. PML is caused by reactivation of the JC polyoma virus in the setting of immunosuppression. Subsequently, a study of more than 3000 patients who had received a mean of 17.9 monthly doses of natalizumab was conducted to assess the risk for PML. An independent adjudication committee was able to confirm only the three initial cases of PML and therefore estimated the risk for PML to be 1 case per 1000 patients (0.1%) with a 95% confidence interval of 0.2–2.8 cases per 1000 patients [8]. Recently, natalizumab was reintroduced for clinical use in MS under stringent safety guidelines as a monotherapy. Based on positive induction and long-term maintenance trials in CD, natalizumab has recently been submitted to the FDA for consideration of approval.

Conclusion

Three TNF antagonists (infliximab, adalimumab, and certolizumab pegol) have been shown to be effective for the induction and maintenance of disease control in CD. In the era of biological therapy in IBD, we can begin to restate our treatment goals to include inducing and maintaining remission, promoting mucosal healing, preventing complications, improving quality of life, and reducing the need for surgery and hospitalization. Emerging data suggest that these goals may best be achieved by the use of infliximab and other anti-TNF agents early in the disease process. However, efficacy and toxicity need to be balanced. To advocate TNF blockade early in disease, there is a pressing need for reliable biomarkers that will adequately predict who will respond to therapy and who will develop complications if left untreated. The addition of newer anti-TNF agents to our armamentarium will ultimately provide choices for patients and physicians, and provide important options if one TNF inhibitor ceases to work. With reports of rare but serious side effects in patients on combination immunomodulators and biological treatments, the risk–benefit of concomitant immunosuppressive therapy has recently been questioned. The clinical significance of immunogenicity and relative immunogenicity between biological treatment options is not yet known. Newer agents that target different aspects of inflammation are also needed, as in the most successful of studies TNF inhibition is effective long term in no more than 40% of patients.

Biological agents in IBD: indications, route of administration, and dosages

	Indications	Route of administration	Induction dose	Loading dose	Maintenance dose
Infliximab	Reduction of: • signs and symptoms, and inducing and maintaining remission in adult and paediatric patients with CD and an inadequate response to conventional therapy • the number of fistulas and for maintaining fistula closure in adults with CD • signs and symptoms, inducing and maintaining clinical remission and mucosal healing, and eliminating corticosteroid use in patients with moderately to severely active UC and an inadequate response to conventional therapy	Infusion	5 mg/kg IV at 0, 2, and 6 weeks		5 mg/kg IV q8 weeks
Adalimumab	For reducing signs and symptoms, and inducing and maintaining clinical remission in adult patients with moderately to severely active CD and an adequate response to conventional therapy	Subcutaneous, pre-filled syringe, injectable pen		160 mg at week 0, 80 mg at week 2	40 mg SC every other week or weekly

Biological agents in IBD: indications, route of administration, and dosages (continued)

	Indications	Route of administration	Induction dose	Loading dose	Maintenance dose
	For reducing signs and symptoms, and inducing clinical remission in these patients if they have also lost response to, or are intolerant of, infliximab				
Certolizumab pegol	In development; has demonstrated significant efficacy in phase III studies in CD	Subcutaneous		400 mg SC at weeks 0, 2, and 4	400 mg SC q4 weeks
Natalizumab	For inducing and maintaining clinical response and remission in adult patients with moderately to severely active CD with evidence of inflammation and an inadequate response to, or unable to tolerate, conventional CD therapies and inhibitors of TNFα	Intravenous	300 mg IV at weeks 0 and 4 (in patients with raised CRP levels)		300 mg IV q4 weeks

Major clinical trials with biologics in IBD

Drug	Study name	Reference	Indication	Aim of study
Infliximab		Targan et al., N Engl J Med 1997; **337**: 1029–35	CD	Induction
		Present et al., N Engl J Med 1999; **340**: 1398–405	CD – fistulas	Induction
	ACCENT I	Rutgeerts et al., Gastroenterology 1999; **117**: 761–9	CD	Maintenance
	ACCENT II	Hanauer et al., Lancet 2002; **359**: 1541–9	CD	Maintenance
		Sands et al., N Engl J Med 2004; **350**: 876–85	CD – fistulas	Maintenance
		Lichtenstein et al. Gastroenterology 2005; **128**: 862–9		
	REACH	Hyams et al., Gastroenterology 2007; **132**: 863–73	CD – paediatric	Induction and maintenance
	ACT1 and ACT2	Rutgeerts et al., N Engl J Med 2005; **353**: 2462–7	UC	Induction and maintenance
Adalimumab	CLASSIC I	Hanauer et al., Gastroenterology 2006; **130**: 323–33	CD	Induction
	CLASSIC II	Sandborn et al., Gut 2007; **56**: 1232–9	CD	Maintenance
	CHARM	Colombel et al., Gastroenterology 2007; **132**: 52–65	CD	Maintenance
Certolizumab pegol	PRECiSE 1	Schreiber et al., Gastroenterology 2005; **129**: 807–18	CD	Induction
		Sandborn et al., N Engl J Med 2007; **357**: 228–38	CD	Induction and maintenance
	PRECiSE 2	Schreiber et al., N Engl J Med 2007; **357**: 239–50	CD	Maintenance
Natalizumab	ENACT 1	Ghosh et al., N Engl J Med 2003; **348**: 68–72	CD	Induction
	ENCORE	Sandborn et al., N Engl J Med 2005; **353**: 1912–25	CD	Induction
		Targan et al., Gastroenterology 2007; **132**: 1672–83	CD – high baseline CRP	Induction
	ENACT 2	Sandborn et al., N Engl J Med 2005; **353**: 1912–25	CD	Maintenance

References

1 Munkholm P. Review article: the incidence and prevalence of colorectal cancer in inflammatory bowel disease. *Aliment Pharmacol Ther* 2003; **18**(Suppl 2): 1–5.
2 Strober W, Fuss IJ, and Blumberg RS. The immunology of mucosal models of inflammation. *Annu Rev Immunol* 2002; **20**: 495–549.
3 Judge TA and Lichstenstein GR. Inflammatory bowel disease. In: Friedman SL, McQuaid KR, and Grendell JH (eds) *Current Diagnosis and Treatment in Gastroenterology*, 2nd edn, pp. 108–130. New York: Lange Medical Books/McGraw Hill, 2003.
4 Hommes D, *et al.* Digestive Disease Week 2006 (Abstract 749).
5 D'Haens GR, *et al.* Digestive Disease Week 2006 (Abstract 764).
6 Sandborn WJ, Colombel JF, Enns R, *et al*; International Efficacy of Natalizumab as Active Crohn's Therapy (ENACT-1) Trial Group; Evaluation of Natalizumab as Continuous Therapy (ENACT-2) Trial Group. Natalizumab induction and maintenance therapy for Crohn's disease. *N Engl J Med* 2005; **353**: 1912–25.
7 Targan SR, *et al.* Digestive Disease Week 2006 (Abstract 747).
8 Yousry TA, Major EO, Ryschkewitsch C, *et al.* Evaluation of patients treated with natalizumab for progressive multifocal leukoencephalopathy. *N Engl J Med* 2006; **354**: 924–33.

Adalimumab (Humira)

Chemical properties	Recombinant human IgG1 monoclonal antibody, 148 kDa
Manufacture	Produced in Chinese Hamster Ovary cells
Stability	Stable for at least 24 months if stored in the dark at 2–8°C
Pharmacokinetics	After a single 40-mg subcutaneous injection, average peak serum concentration was 4.7 µg/ml after 5.4 days. Average bioavailability compared with intravenous dosing is 64%. Half-life 10–20 days
Metabolism	Thought to be catabolized in a similar manner to normal human immunoglobulin. In patients receiving adalimumab monotherapy, clearance in patients with RA is faster than in those with moderate to severe psoriasis
Drug interactions	Methotrexate, azathioprine, and 6-mercaptopurine probably decrease clearance rate of adalimumab, although this does not appear to be dose dependent

Clinical trial data – Crohn's disease

Moderate to severely active luminal Crohn's disease

Study 1 – CLASSIC 1, Phase II/III study [1] The CLASSIC I trial was a randomized, double-blind, placebo-controlled, dose-ranging study performed to evaluate the efficacy of adalimumab induction therapy in 299 patients with moderate to severe Crohn's disease (CDAI 220–450). All of the patients enrolled in this study had had CD for at least 4 months and were naive to TNF antagonists. Patients were randomized to receive one of four dosing regimens: placebo subcutaneously at weeks 0 and 2; adalimumab 40 mg subcutaneously at week 0 and 20 mg at week 2; adalimumab 80 mg at week 0 and 40 mg at week 2; or adalimumab 160 mg at week 0 and 80 mg at week 2. Patients were followed for 4 weeks. The primary endpoint was the rate of remission (CDAI <150) at week 4. Secondary endpoints included proportion of patients with a 70- and 100-point decrease from baseline in CDAI.

There was a linear dose–response across the three adalimumab groups at week 4 for the primary endpoint of remission. The rates of remission at week

4 were 18%, 24%, and 36% in patients who received induction therapy with adalimumab 40/20, 80/40, and 160/80 mg, respectively, compared with 12% in patients who received placebo. The differences in remission rates were statistically significant between patients who received induction therapy with the highest doses of adalimumab (160/80 mg) and those who received placebo ($P < 0.05$). The percentage of patients with a 70-point decrease from baseline in CDAI scores was significantly higher in all three active treatment arms when compared with the placebo arm ($P < 0.05$ for each comparison) [1].

CLASSIC I

Treatment	Response (4weeks)		Remission (4 weeks)* CDAI ≤ 150
	ΔCDAI 70	ΔCDAI 100	
Adalimumab			
40 mg/20 mg	54%	34%	18%
80 mg/40 mg	40%	40%	24%
160 mg/80 mg	50%	50%	36%
Placebo	37%	25%	12%

*Primary endpoint: adalimumab 40/20 mg vs placebo, $P = 0.36$; 80/40mg vs placebo, $P = 0.06$; 160/80mg vs placebo, $P = 0.001$.

Study 2 – CHARM, Phase II/III study [2] Maintenance of clinical response in Crohn's disease. Maintenance therapy with adalimumab for the treatment of CD was evaluated in the multicentre, double-blind, placebo-controlled 56-week CHARM study. Some 854 patients received open-label induction with adalimumab 80 mg subcutaneously at week 0 and 40 mg at week 2. 499 primary responders (defined as decrease in CDAI ≥70 points from baseline) at week 4 were randomized to placebo, adalimumab 40 mg every other week, or adalimumab 40 mg weekly through week 56.

Approximately 50% of the patients enrolled in the CHARM study had received prior treatment with TNF antagonists. Steroid tapering was permitted after week 8 for patients who achieved a clinical response. The co-primary endpoints of the study were remission (CDAI <150) at week 26 and week 56 in the randomized responder population.

Throughout follow-up, patients who responded to initial induction therapy with adalimumab by week 4 and who continued to receive maintenance therapy with adalimumab showed a greater therapeutic benefit than responders to induction therapy, who were subsequently randomized to maintenance with placebo. At week 26, the proportion of patients who achieved clinical remission was higher in patients who received adalimumab 40 mg every other week and 40 mg weekly (40% and 47%, respectively) than patients who received placebo (17%, $P<0.001$ vs placebo for both comparisons). At week 56, remission rates were still significantly higher among patients receiving active treatment in comparison with the placebo group ($P<0.001$ for both active treatment arms vs placebo). At week 26, the percentage of patients who achieved steroid-free remission (defined as off steroids for 3 months or more) while receiving adalimumab (35% and 30% for adalimumab every other week and every week, respectively) were also higher when compared with the rate of steroid-free remission in the placebo group (3%, $P<0.001$). Steroid-free remission rates were still significantly higher at week 56 compared with those in the placebo group.

As a subanalysis in CHARM, maintenance of complete healing of draining fistulas was assessed at weeks 26 and 56 in a subgroup of 117 patients who had active enterocutaneous fistulas at both screening and baseline. The proportion of patients with completely healed fistulas at week 26 was higher in patients who received adalimumab (30% adalimumab maintenance vs 13% placebo maintenance; $P=0.043$ for the pre-specified secondary endpoint). Maintenance of remission with adalimumab was efficacious in patients compared with placebo irrespective of whether patients were previously exposed to an anti-TNF agent or immunomodulators [2].

CHARM

Treatment	Response (week 26/56)		Remission (week 26/56)*
	ΔCDAI 70	ΔCDAI 100	CDAI$\leq$150
Adalimumab			
40 mg e.o.w.	54%/43%	52%/41%	40%/36%
40 mg/week	56%/49%	52%/48%	47%/41%
Placebo	28%/18%	26%/16%	17%/12%

*Primary endpoint. The percentage of randomized responders in remission was significantly greater in the adalimumab 40-mg every other week (e.o.w.) and 40-mg/week groups vs placebo at week 26 ($P<0.001$) and week 56 ($P<0.001$). There were no significant differences in efficacy between the adalimumab e.o.w. and weekly groups.

Study 3 – The GAIN Induction Study, Phase II/II trial [3] The GAIN study specifically addressed efficacy of adalimumab for induction of remission in 325 patients with moderate to severe CD who had secondary failure to infliximab therapy (loss of response, development of intolerance to the drug, or both). Approximately 59% of the patients who entered into the GAIN Study had had a previous adverse reaction to infliximab, and 51% had loss of response to the drug. Approximately 12% of patients had both an adverse reaction and lost responsiveness to infliximab. Patients were randomized to receive placebo or adalimumab 160 mg subcutaneously at week 0 and 80 mg at week 2. The primary endpoint was remission (CDAI <150) at week 4. Secondary endpoints included a 70–100-point decrease in CDAI scores from baseline at week 4.

A significantly higher percentage of patients who received adalimumab 160 mg at week 0 and 80 mg at week 2 were in remission at week 4 (21% vs 7%, $P < 0.001$). Likewise, significant differences in clinical responses (defined as decreases in CDAI of 70 and 100 points) were seen in the adalimumab group compared with placebo. Clinical benefit was demonstrated following adalimumab administration as early as week 2. Response and remission was seen across subgroups and did not depend on whether patients had lost response to infliximab or had an adverse event [3].

GAIN Study

Treatment	Response (4 weeks)		Remission (4 weeks)*
	ΔCDAI 70	ΔCDAI 100	CDAI$\leq$150
Adalimumab			
160 mg/80 mg	52%	38%	21%
Placebo	34%	25%	7%

*Primary endpoint; $P < 0.001$ adalimumab vs placebo in patients who had responded to another anti-TNF agent and then lost that response or were intolerant of the agent.

References

1 Hanauer SB, Sandborn WJ, Rutgeerts P, et al. Human anti-tumor necrosis factor monoclonal antibody (adalimumab) in Crohn's disease: the CLASSIC-I trial. *Gastroenterology* 2006; **130**: 323–33.

2 Colombel JF, Sandborn WJ, Rutgeerts P, et al. Adalimumab for maintenance of clinical response and remission in patients with Crohn's disease: the CHARM trial. *Gastroenterology* 2007; **132**: 52–65.

3 Sandborn WJ, Rutgeerts P, Enns R, et al. Adalimumab induction therapy for Crohn disease previously treated with infliximab: a randomized trial. *Ann Intern Med* 2007; **146**: 829–38.

Infliximab (Remicade)

Administration	Intravenous infusion in normal saline (sodium chloride 0.9%) over 2 hours
Chemical properties	Recombinant human–murine chimaeric IgG1 monoclonal antibody
Manufacture	Produced in the cell line by continuous perfusion
Stability	Stable for at least 36 months if stored in the dark at 2–8°C
Pharmacokinetics	Single dose of 5 mg/kg in Crohn's disease indicates median terminal half-life of 8–9.5 days. Single 3–20-mg/kg IV dosing shows a linear dose range, and a blood level relationship indicating mainly intravascular department distribution. Eight weeks after a dose given during scheduled maintenance therapy, stable blood levels of approximately 0.5–6 µg/ml were seen, with no systemic accumulation of drug. The development of antibodies against infliximab increases clearance
Metabolism	Thought to be metabolized in a manner similar to that of normal human immunoglobulin, hence a similar half-life
Drug interactions	Azathioprine, 6-mercaptopurine, and methotrexate probably decrease the formation of antibodies against infliximab and increase plasma concentrations of infliximab

Clinical trial data – Crohn's disease

Moderate to severely active luminal Crohn's disease

Phase II/III trial [1] A short-term study of chimaeric monoclonal antibody cA2 to TNFα for CD. This was a 12-week, multicentre, double-blind, placebo-controlled trial of cA2 in 100 patients with moderate to severe CD resistant to conventional medical therapies. All patients had CDAI scores between 220 and 400. Patients were randomly assigned to receive a single 2-hour intravenous infusion of either placebo or infliximab at 5, 10, or 20 mg/kg. Clinical response was defined as reduction of 70 or more points in the CDAI at 4 weeks.

Secondary endpoints included a 100-point decrease in the CDAI and clinical remission.

A dose–response was not demonstrated in this study; in fact, the 5-mg/kg dose appeared to be superior to the higher doses.

Treatment	Clinical response (week 4)
Infliximab	
5 mg/kg	81%
10 mg/kg	50%
20 mg/kg	64%
Placebo	17%

At 4 weeks, 33% of the infliximab-treated group were in remission, compared with 4% of the placebo group ($P=0.005$). Approximately half of the patients who had a clinical response at either 2 or 4 weeks also entered remission. Clinical response with infliximab also correlated with decreases in C-reactive protein (CRP) levels and improvements in the IBD questionnaire, an IBD-specific quality-of-life index. Responses appeared to persist through 12 weeks, with an overall response rate at 12 weeks after a single infusion of infliximab of 41%, compared with 12% in the placebo group ($P=0.008$) [1].

Phase II study – Targan et al. [1]

Treatment	Response (week 4)* ΔCDAI 70	Remission (week 4) CDAI ≤150
Infliximab		
5 mg/kg	81%	48%
10 mg/kg	50%	25%
20 mg/kg	64%	25%
Placebo	17%	4%

*Primary endpoint. Response: $P<0.001$ combined infliximab vs placebo. Remission: $P=0.005$ combined infliximab vs placebo.

ACCENT I, Phase II/III study [2] A multicentre, randomized, double-blind, placebo-controlled trial that evaluated maintenance therapy in infliximab in patients with moderately to severely active luminal CD who responded to a single infusion of infliximab. Some 573 patients with active CD who responded to a single infusion of infliximab at week 0 were randomized to receive placebo at weeks 2 and 6, then every 8 weeks; or infliximab 5 mg/kg at weeks 2 and 6, and then either 5 or 10 mg/kg every 8 weeks. 58% of the 573 original patients responded to infliximab at week 2 (decrease in CDAI ≥ 70 from baseline and improvement in score ≥ 25%). The pre-specified co-primary endpoints were the proportion of patients who responded at week 2 and were in remission (CDAI <150) at week 30 and the time to loss of response up to week 54 in patients who responded.

At week 30, 21% of patients randomized to placebo were in remission, compared with 39% of those treated with infliximab 5 mg/kg and 45% of patients treated with 10 mg/kg every 8 weeks. The median time to loss of response was 38 weeks (5 mg/kg infliximab) and more than 54 weeks (10 mg/kg infliximab) for patients randomized to scheduled maintenance infliximab, compared with 19 weeks for patients treated with a single dose of infliximab and then randomized to placebo. In this study, about three times as many patients treated with scheduled maintenance infliximab had discontinued corticosteroids while in clinical remission compared with patients who received a single dose of infliximab and were randomized to placebo (29% vs 9%) [2].

ACCENT I – Phase III study

Treatment	Remission (week 30)* CDAI ≤ 150	Median time to loss of response (week 54)*
Infliximab		
5 mg/kg	39%	38 weeks
10 mg/kg	45%	54 weeks
Placebo	21%	19 weeks

*Co-primary endpoints. At week 30, Remission: 5 mg/kg vs placebo ($P=0.003$); 10 mg/kg vs placebo ($P=0.0002$). Patients in the infliximab groups combined were more likely to sustain clinical remission than those receiving placebo (odds ratio 2.7, 95% CI 1.6–4.6). Throughout the 54-week trial, median time to loss of response for 5-mg/kg group vs placebo, $P=0.002$, and for 10-mg/kg vs placebo, $P=0.0002$.

Subsequently, a substudy performed during ACCENT I revealed that patients treated with scheduled infliximab therapy compared with patients receiving a single infusion then were randomized to placebo (but were allowed to receive subsequent infliximab open-label for the development of symptoms) achieved mucosal healing. Baseline ileocolonoscopy was performed on 99 patients. Mucosal ulceration was present at baseline in 82%. Of these patients, 74 and 58 underwent follow-up endoscopic examination at weeks 10 and 54, respectively.

At week 10, 29% of patients in the scheduled infliximab maintenance group (who received three doses of infliximab 5 mg/kg on weeks 0, 2, and 6) showed mucosal healing, compared with 3% of patients in the group who received a single infusion at week 0 ($P=0.0006$). At week 54, a significantly higher proportion of patients in the scheduled treatment strategy group demonstrated mucosal healing compared with patients who received infliximab episodically (44% vs 18%, $P=0.041$) [3].

ACT 1 and ACT 2 [3]

Treatment	Response (week 8) (ACT 1/ACT 2)* ΔMayo score 3 points and ≥30%	Remission (week 8) (ACT 1/ACT 2) Mayo score ≤2
Infliximab		
5 mg/kg	69%/64%	39%/34%
10 mg/kg	62%/69%	32%/28%
Placebo	37%/29%	15%/6%

*Primary endpoint. Response at week 8 in ACT 1 and ACT 2, infliximab vs placebo: $P<0.001$ for both comparisons. In both studies, patients who received infliximab were more likely to have a clinical response at week 30 ($P \leq 0.002$ for all comparisons).

Fistulizing Crohn's disease

Infliximab in Crohn's disease with enterocutaneous fistulas – Phase II study [4] This randomized, placebo-controlled, double-blind, multicentre study of infliximab for the treatment of fistulas in patients with CD included 94 adult patients who had draining abdominal or perianal fistulas of at least 3 months' duration as complications of CD. Patients were randomly assigned to receive either placebo, 5 mg/kg infliximab, or 10 mg/kg infliximab administered intravenously at weeks 0, 2, and 6. The primary endpoint was a reduction of 50% or more from baseline in the number of draining fistulas observed at two or more consecutive study visits. The secondary endpoint was the closure of all fistulas.

Some 68% of patients receiving 5 mg/kg infliximab and 56% of those receiving 10 mg/kg achieved the primary endpoint, compared with 26% of patients in the placebo group ($P=0.002$ and $P=0.02$, respectively). In addition, 55% of patients who received 5 mg/kg infliximab and 38% of those who received 10 mg/kg had closure of all fistulas, compared with 13% of patients in the placebo group ($P=0.001$ and $P=0.04$, respectively). The median length of time that fistulas remained closed was 3 months [4].

Treatment	Fistula healing* (reduction of ≥50%)	Complete fistula response (no draining fistulas on ≥2 consecutive visits)
Infliximab		
5 mg/kg	68%	55%
10 mg/kg	56%	38%
Placebo	26%	13%

*Primary endpoint. Significant fistula healing was demonstrated in the 5- and 10-mg/kg infliximab groups vs placebo ($P=0.002$ and $P=0.02$, respectively). In addition, complete fistula closure was demonstrated in the 5- and 10-mg/kg infliximab groups vs placebo $P=0.001$ and $P=0.04$, respectively).

ACCENT II – infliximab maintenance therapy for fistulizing CD [5]

ACCENT II was a multicentre, randomized, double-blind, placebo-controlled trial that evaluated the efficacy of infliximab maintenance therapy in 306 adult patients with CD who had one or more draining abdominal or perianal fistulas. Of 306 patients enrolled, 282 received 5 mg/kg infliximab at weeks 0, 2, and 6, and were available for randomization at week 14. At week 14, responders (defined as a reduction of 50% from baseline in the number of draining fistulas at both weeks 10 and 14) were randomized to receive placebo or infliximab 5 mg/kg every 8 weeks, and followed until week 54. Of 195 patients with a response at week 14, 99 were randomly assigned to receive placebo and 96 patients received infliximab maintenance.

Of patients randomized to receive infliximab maintenance, 36% had complete fistula closure at week 54 compared with 19% of patients receiving placebo ($P=0.009$). The time to loss of response was significantly longer for patients who received infliximab maintenance therapy than for those who received placebo (>40 vs 14 weeks; $P=0.001$) [5].

ACCENT II

Treatment	Complete fistula response (week 54) (absence of draining fistulas)	Time to loss of response*
Infliximab 5 mg/kg	36%	>40 weeks
Placebo	19%	14 weeks

*Primary endpoint. The time to loss of response was significantly longer for patients receiving infliximab maintenance therapy than for those in the placebo group ($P<0.001$). At week 54, fewer patients in the placebo group had a complete absence of draining fistulas compared with the infliximab maintenance group ($P=0.009$).

The effect of infliximab maintenance on hospitalizations, surgeries, and Crohn's disease-related procedures was evaluated retrospectively in ACCENT II. The rate of hospitalization per 100 patients was significantly lower in patients who received infliximab maintenance than those who received placebo (14% vs 31%; $P < 0.05$). The mean number of inpatient surgeries and procedures per 100 patients in the infliximab maintenance group was reduced by over 70% compared with placebo maintenance ($P < 0.001$) [6].

Paediatric Crohn's disease

The REACH study [7] The REACH study was a multicentre, randomized, open-label study designed to evaluate the efficacy and safety of maintenance with infliximab in children with moderately to severely active CD, defined as a paediatric CDAI of > 30 points. Some 112 patients underwent induction therapy with infliximab 5 mg/kg at weeks 0, 2, and 6. Patients responding at week 10 were randomized to receive maintenance with infliximab 5 mg/kg every 8 weeks or every 12 weeks through week 46, and were followed through week 54. At week 54, the rates of clinical response and remission were significantly higher in patients who received infliximab every 8 weeks (63.5% and 55.8%, respectively) than in patients who received infliximab 5 mg/kg every 12 weeks (33% and 23.5%, respectively ($P \leq 0.002$ for both comparisons). At week 10, 88.4% of patients responded to infliximab and 58.9% achieved clinical remission [7].

REACH

Treatment	Response (week 30/54) ΔPCDAI $\geq$ 15 and total score $\leq$ 30	Remission (week 30/54) PCDAI $\leq$ 10
5 mg/kg q12 weeks	47%/33%	35%/24%
5 mg/kg q8 weeks	73%/64%	60%/56%

At week 54, response and remission in patients receiving infliximab every 8 weeks vs every 12 weeks, $P = 0.002$ and $P < 0.001$, respectively.

Ulcerative colitis

ACT 1 and ACT 2 [8] FDA approval for the treatment of UC was based on the results of two large-scale, randomized, double-blind, placebo-controlled, multicentre clinical studies, the 54-week ACT 1 and the 30-week ACT 2 trials. The ACT trials were conducted and published simultaneously, and investigated infliximab in patients with active UC who had failed steroids or other conventional treatments. The inclusion criteria in the studies were the same, except that in ACT 2 25% of patients who had failed 5-ASA alone were enrolled. Otherwise, in both ACT 1 and ACT 2, inclusion criteria were active UC (defined as a Mayo Clinical Disease Activity (MCAI) score of 6–12) despite the use of steroids alone or in combination with 6-mercaptopurine or azathioprine. Endoscopic evidence of moderate or severe UC had to be demonstrated (Mayo endoscopic subscore 2).

Amongst 728 patients enrolled in the two studies, 72% were treated with concomitant 5-ASA, 56% with corticosteroids, and 46% with 6-mercaptopurine–azathioprine. Doses of concomitant medications remained constant except for corticosteroids, which were tapered by 5 mg weekly after week 8 until a dose of 20 mg daily was reached. Thereafter, the dose was reduced by 2.5 mg weekly until discontinuation. The primary endpoint was clinical response at week 8, defined as a decrease in the Mayo score of at least 30% and at least 3 points, plus a decrease in the rectal bleeding score of at least 1 or a rectal bleeding score of 0 or 1. Secondary endpoints were remission at week 8 defined as a Mayo score ≤ 2 with no individual subscores > 1, mucosal healing at week 8, endoscopic subscore 0 or 1, and response, remission, and mucosal healing at weeks 30 and 54.

In each study, 364 patients with moderate to severe active UC received either placebo or infliximab 5 mg/kg intravenously at weeks 0, 2, and 6, and then every 8 weeks through week 46 in ACT 1 or week 22 in ACT 2. In ACT 1, 69% of patients who received 5 mg/kg infliximab and 61% of those who received 10 mg/kg infliximab had a clinical response at week 8, compared with 37% in the placebo group ($P < 0.001$ for both comparisons). In ACT 2, 64% of patients receiving 5 mg/kg and 69% of those receiving 10 mg/kg had a clinical response at week 8, compared with 29% in the placebo group ($P \leq 0.001$ for both comparisons). In both studies, patients who received infliximab were more likely to have a clinical response at week 30 ($P \leq 0.002$ for all comparisons). At 8, 30, and 54 weeks there were statistically significant differences in clinical remission in patients treated with infliximab 5 or 10 mg/kg every 8 weeks compared with placebo. Overall, there was a remission rate in the infliximab maintenance groups of 2 to 2.5 times that seen with placebo ($P \leq 0.003$ for all comparisons). Infliximab maintenance allowed reductions in the median daily steroid dose. A higher percentage of patients demonstrated mucosal healing in the infliximab maintenance group compared with placebo ($P < 0.001$ for all comparisons; at weeks 30 and 54 ($P \leq 0.009$ for all comparisons) [8].

References

1 Targan SR, Hanauer SB, van Deventer SJ, *et al.* A short-term study of chimeric monoclonal antibody cA2 to tumor necrosis factor alpha for Crohn's disease. Crohn's Disease cA2 Study Group. *N Engl J Med* 1997; **337**: 1029–35.

2 Hanauer SB, Feagan BG, Lichtenstein GR, *et al.* Maintenance infliximab for Crohn's disease: the ACCENT I randomised trial. *Lancet* 2002; **359**: 1541–49.

3 Rutgeerts P, Feagan BG, Lichtenstein GR, *et al.* Comparison of scheduled and episodic treatment strategies of infliximab in Crohn's disease. *Gastroenterology* 2004; **126**: 402–13.

4 Present DH, Rutgeerts P, Targan S, *et al.* Infliximab for the treatment of fistulas in patients with Crohn's disease. *N Engl J Med* 1999; **340**: 1398–405.

5 Sands BE, Anderson FH, Bernstein CN, *et al*. Infliximab maintenance therapy for fistulizing Crohn's disease. *N Engl J Med* 2004; **350**: 876–85.

6 Lichtenstein GR, Yan S, Bala M, Blank M, and Sands BE. Infliximab maintenance treatment reduces hospitalizations, surgeries, and procedures in fistulizing Crohn's disease. *Gastroenterology* 2005; **128**: 862–9.

7 Hyams J, Crandall W, Kugathasan S, *et al*. Induction and maintenance infliximab therapy for the treatment of moderate-to-severe Crohn's disease in children. *Gastroenterology* 2007; **132**: 863–73.

8 Rutgeerts P, Sandborn WJ, Feagan BG, *et al*. Infliximab for induction and maintenance therapy for ulcerative colitis. *N Engl J Med* 2005; **353**: 2462–76.

9 Lichtenstein GR, Feagan BG, Cohen RD, *et al*. Serious infections and mortality in association with therapies for Crohn's disease: TREAT registry. *Clin Gastroenterol Hepatol* 2006; **4**: 621–30.

Natalizumab (Tysabri)

Chemical properties	Recombinant humanized IgG4 kappa monoclonal antibody. Natalizumab contains human framework regions and the complentarity determining regions of the murine antibody that binds the α4 integrin. Molecular weight 149 kDa.
Manufacture	Produced in murine myeloma cells
Stability	Lyophilized single-use vials are stable when stored refrigerated at 2–8°C. Once reconstituted, natalizumab must be used within 8 hours
Pharmacokinetics	Following repeat intravenous administration of a 300-mg dose of natalizumab to patients with MS, the mean maximum observed curate serum concentration was 110 ± 52 µg/ml. The observed time to steady state was approximately 24 weeks after every 4 weeks of dosing. The mean half-life is 11 ± 4 days.
Drug interactions	The presence of persistent anti-natalizumab antibodies increases natalizumab clearance by approximately 3-fold. Given the side-effect profile, natalizumab is recommended for use only as monotherapy

Clinical trial data – Crohn's disease

Moderate to severely active Crohn's disease

Natalizumab for active Crohn's disease – Phase II/III study Natalizumab Pan-European Study Group. This was a double-blind, placebo-controlled trial of natalizumab in 248 patients with moderate to severe CD (CDAI 220–450). Patients were randomly assigned to receive one of four treatments: two infusions of placebo, one infusion of 3 mg/kg natalizumab followed by placebo, two infusions of 3 mg/kg natalizumab, or two infusions of 6 mg/kg natalizumab given 4 weeks apart. The primary efficacy endpoint was clinical remission defined by a score of CDAI <150 at week 6, and clinical response defined as a decrease in the CDAI of at least 70 points in the highest dose of natalizumab utilized. All other efficacy analyses were pre-specified as secondary endpoints.

The study did not attain its primary endpoint in that the group given two infusions of 6 mg/kg natalizumab did not have a significantly higher rate of clinical remission than the placebo group at week 6. However, both groups that had received two infusions of natalizumab had higher remission rates than the placebo group at multiple time points. Natalizumab also produced significant improvement in response rates [1].

Treatment	Response (week 6) ΔCDAI 70	Remission (week 6)* CDAI ≤ 150
Natalizumab		
3 mg/kg	59%	29%
3 mg/kg q4 weeks (×2)	71%	44%
6 mg/kg q4 weeks (×2)	57%	31%
Placebo	38%	27%

*Primary endpoint; P not significant at primary endpoint. However, both groups that received two infusions of natalizumab had higher remission rates than the placebo group at multiple other time points.

ENACT 1 – Phase III [2] ENACT 1 was a phase III, international, randomized, double-blind, placebo-controlled trial to assess induction of response in remission compared with placebo in patients with active CD treated with natalizumab. The study population consisted of patients with moderately to severely active CD (CDAI 220–450). Some 905 patients were randomized 4:1 to natalizumab 300 mg or placebo with one infusion every 4 weeks. The primary endpoints were clinical response at week 10 defined as a 70-point decrease from baseline CDAI score, with a contingent primary endpoint being remission at week 10 (CDAI <150).

At the week 10 primary endpoint, the natalizumab and placebo groups had similar rates of response (56% and 49%, respectively; $P=0.005$) and remission (37% and 30%, respectively; $P=0.12$). In patients who had a raised CRP level at baseline (upper limit of normal 2.87 mg/l), in patients with active disease despite the use of immunosuppressants, and in patients who had previously received anti-TNF therapy, each subgroup was significantly more likely to have response or remission after treatment with natalizumab than after receiving placebo at week 10 [2].

ENACT 1

Treatment	Response (10 weeks)* ΔCDAI 70	Remission (10 weeks) CDAI ≤ 150
Natalizumab		
300 mg q4 weeks	56%	37%
Placebo	49%	30%

*Primary endpoint; $P=0.051$ for response, $P=0.12$ for remission at 10 weeks.

ENCORE study – Phase III [3] ENCORE was an international, randomized, double-placebo-controlled trial to assess induction of clinical response and remission in patients with moderately to severely active CD (CDAI 220–450) and raised serum CRP levels (2.87 mg/l). Patients were randomized 1:1 to natalizumab 300 mg ($n=259$) or placebo ($n=250$) for one infusion every 4 weeks. The primary endpoint was clinical response (70-point decrease from baseline CDAI) by week 8 that was sustained through week 12. The contingent primary endpoint was remission (CDAI <150) at week 8 that was sustained through week 12.

Some 48% of natalizumab-treated patients had a response at week 8 that was sustained through week 12, compared with 32% of placebo-treated patients ($P<0.001$). There was a statistically significant difference in response rates between the natalizumab and placebo groups at weeks 4, 8, and 12 ($P \leq 0.001$ for all comparisons). Some 26% of natalizumab-treated patients demonstrated sustained remission from week 8 to 12, versus 16% in the placebo group ($P=0.002$) [3].

ENCORE

Treatment	Response (weeks 8, 12, 8 + 12)		Remission (weeks 8, 12, 8 + 12) CDAI ≤ 150
	ΔCDAI 70*	ΔCDAI 100	
Natalizumab			
300 mg q4 weeks	56%/60%/48%	48%/49%/39%	32%/38%/26%
Placebo	40%/44%/32%	33%/31%/22%	21%/25%/16%

*Primary endpoint. All patients with raised baseline CRP levels; response at week 8 sustained through week 12 occurred in 48% of natalizumab-treated patients and 32% of patients receiving placebo ($P<0.001$).
Sustained remission occurred in 26% of natalizumab-treated patients and 16% of those receiving placebo ($P=0.002$).

ENACT 2 – Phase III [2] ENACT 2 was an international, randomized, double-blind, placebo-controlled trial to assess the efficacy of natalizumab maintenance in patients who were induced into response with natalizumab. The study population consisted of patients who had responded to natalizumab (70-point or greater decrease in CDAI from baseline) and had completed the ENACT 1 induction trial. Some 339 patients were randomized 1:1 to receive natalizumab 300 mg IV every 4 weeks for a total of 12 infusions or placebo, one infusion every 4 weeks for 12 infusions. The primary endpoint was sustained clinical response for six continuous months (up to 9 months after initiation of natalizumab). The secondary endpoints were remission (CDAI <150) for 6 months, and the percentage of patients discontinuing steroids at 6 months.

Maintenance natalizumab resulted in higher rates of sustained response (61% vs 28%, $P < 0.001$) and remission (44% vs 26%, $P = 0.003$) through week 36 vs placebo. The rates of sustained response in remission were significantly higher in the natalizumab group at every point, beginning at week 20 and continuing through week 60. Sustained response rates at week 60 were 54% in the natalizumab group versus 20% in the placebo group ($P < 0.001$). Sustained remission at week 60 was 39% in the natalizumab group compared with 15% in the placebo group ($P < 0.001$). At week 30, corticosteroid-free remission was demonstrated in 45% of natalizumab-treated patients versus 22% of placebo-treated patients ($P = 0.003$). This difference was sustained through week 60 [2].

ENACT 2

Treatment	Sustained response (week 36/60)* ΔCDAI 70	Sustained remission (week 36/60) CDAI ≤ 150
Natalizumab		
300 mg q4 weeks	67%/59%	55%/55%
Placebo	37%/24%	30%/22%

*Primary endpoint. Continuing natalizumab resulted in higher rates of sustained response ($P < 0.001$) and remission ($P = 0.03$) through week 36 than did switching to placebo.

Natalizumab and progressive multifocal leucoencephalopathy

Natalizumab was originally approved by the FDA for the treatment of relapsing forms of MS in November 2004. Because of the occurrence of PML, the use natalizumab was suspended on 28 February 2005. There were three reports of PML in two patients with MS who were also receiving interferon β and in one patient with CD and prior exposure to azathioprine [4]. PML is caused by reactivation of the JC polyoma virus in the setting of immunosuppression. Subsequently, a study of 3417 patients who had recently received natalizumab while participating in clinical trials was undertaken; 3116 patients who had been exposed to a mean of 17.9 monthly doses underwent evaluation for PML. Of these, 44 patients were referred to an expert independent adjudication panel because of clinical findings of possible PML, abnormalities on magnetic resonance imaging (MRI), or a high plasma viral load of JC virus. No patient had detectable JC virus in the cerebrospinal fluid (CSF). PML was ruled out in 43 of the 44 patients, but could not be ruled out in one patient because data on CSF testing and follow-up MRI were not available. Therefore, only the three previously reported cases of PML were confirmed, 1 per 1000 patients treated (95% CI 0.2–2.8 per 1000) [5].

References

1 Ghosh S, Goldin E, Gordon FH, *et al*. Natalizumab for active Crohn's disease. *N Engl J Med* 2003; **348**: 24–32.
2 Sandborn WJ, Colombel JF, Enns R, *et al*. Natalizumab induction and maintenance therapy for Crohn's disease. *N Engl J Med* 2005; **353**: 1912–25.
3 Targan SR, Feagan BG, Fedorak RN, *et al*. Natalizumab for the treatment of active Crohn's disease: results of the ENCORE Trial. *Gastroenterology* 2007; **132**: 1672–83.
4 Kleinschmidt-DeMasters, 2005 #23; Langer-Gould, 2005 #24; Van Assche, 2005 #22. PML is caused by reactivation of the JC polyoma
5 Yousry, 2006 #21

Certolizumab pegol (Cimzia)

Chemical properties	Pegylated humanized Fab' fragment (95% human)
Manufacture	Expressed in *Escherichia coli*
Stability	
Pharmacokinetics	Half-life is 14 days. It is administered subcutaneously and the interval between injections in the pivotal clinical trials was 2–4 weeks
Metabolism	Unclear; however, pegylation is responsible for a prolonged half-life compared with that of a non-pegylated Fab' fragment
Drug interactions	Unclear. Azathioprine, 6-mercaptopurine, and methotrexate probably decrease the clearance rate

Clinical trial data – Crohn's disease

Moderately to severely active luminal Crohn's disease

Phase II study [1] A total of 292 patients with moderately to severely active CD were randomized to receive either placebo or subcutaneous certolizumab pegol (100, 200, or 400 mg) given at weeks 0, 4, and 8. Although patients treated with certolizumab pegol tended toward a clinical response, there were no significant differences between the treatment and placebo groups at the primary endpoint at week 12. In a *post hoc* analysis, it was observed that patients with high baseline CRP levels were more likely to respond. Specifically, amongst patients with a baseline CRP level >10 mg/l, 53% of patients who received certolizumab 400 mg had a clinical response, compared with 18% of patients who received placebo [1].

Phase II

Treatment	Response (week 12) ΔCDAI 100*	Remission (week 12) CDAI ≤ 150
Certolizumab pegol		
100 mg q4 weeks	36%	27%
200 mg q4 weeks	36%	19%
400 mg q4 weeks	44%	26%
Placebo	36%	23%

*Primary endpoint, P not significant (*post hoc* analysis in patients with baseline CRP > 7 mg/l showed significant improvement in the 400-mg group vs placebo).

PRECiSE 1 – Phase III trial [2] PRECiSE 1 was a placebo-controlled phase III trial to evaluate the efficacy and tolerability of subcutaneous certolizumab pegol 400 mg for the induction and maintenance of clinical response and remission in patients with moderately and severely active CD (CDAI 220–450). Some 659 patients were initially randomized to receive placebo ($n=328$) or certolizumab pegol ($n=331$) at week 0 and continued receiving treatment for 26 weeks. Unlike the large maintenance studies of infliximab or adalimumab, this was a placebo-controlled trial without an open-label induction phase. Patients were stratified according to baseline levels of CRP and were randomly assigned to receive either 400 mg certolizumab pegol or placebo subcutaneously at weeks 0, 2, and 4, and then every 4 weeks. Primary endpoints were induction of a response at week 6 (100-point decrease in CDAI) and response at both week 6 and 26.

Results in the intention-to-treat population were similar to those observed in patients with raised CRP levels. A significant difference in response rate was observed as early as week 4 (29% vs 22%, certolizumab pegol vs placebo; $P \leq 0.05$) and the difference in response between the two treatment arms was maintained at week 26 (35% vs 27%, respectively; $P \leq 0.05$). The primary endpoint of sustained clinical response at both weeks 6 and 26 was seen in 23% of certolizumab-treated patients and 16% of those in the placebo group ($P \leq 0.05$) [2].

PRECiSE 1: Phase III

Treatment	Response (ΔCDAI 100)		
	Week 6	Week 26	Weeks 6 and 26*
Certolizumab pegol 400 mg on weeks 0, 2, 4, and q4 weeks	35%	37%	23%
Placebo	27%	27%	16%

*Primary endpoint. In the overall population, response rates at week 6 were 35% in the certolizumab group and 27% in the placebo group ($P=0.02$). At both weeks 6 and 26, the response rates were 23% and 16%, respectively ($P=0.02$). At weeks 6 and 26, the rates of remission in the two groups did not differ significantly ($P=0.17$).

PRECiSE 2 [3] Akin to the pivotal maintenance studies of infliximab and adalimumab in CD, PRECiSE 2 evaluated the efficacy and tolerability of certolizumab pegol for maintenance of clinical response following successful open-label induction in patients with active CD (CDAI 220–450). Some 668 patients underwent open-label induction with certolizumab pegol 400 mg by subcutaneous injection at weeks 0, 2, and 4.

A total of 428 patients (64%) responded to induction (decrease in CDAI of ≥100 points from baseline) at week 6 and were randomized to placebo ($n=212$) or certolizumab pegol 400 mg every 4 weeks ($n=216$) for an additional 20 weeks. Efficacy was evaluated at week 26 using the same criteria for clinical response (decrease of 100 points or more from baseline CDAI).

Clinical response was seen in 63% of patients in the certolizumab pegol group, compared with 36% in the placebo group at week 26 ($P<0.001$), remission (CDAI <150) was achieved by 48% of patients in the certolizumab pegol group compared with 29% in the placebo group ($P<0.001$). In PRECiSE 2, efficacy was demonstrated in patients who were concomitantly taking and/or had previously been exposed to immunomodulators and TNF inhibitors [3].

PRECiSE 2: Phase III

Treatment	Response (week 26) ΔCDAI 100*	Remission (week 26) CDAI ≤ 150
Certolizumab pegol 400 mg q4 weeks	63%	48%
Placebo	36%	29%

*Primary endpoint. Among patients with a response to open-label induction at week 6 (64%), response was maintained through week 26 in 63% of patients in the intention-to-treat population who were receiving certolizumab pegol (vs 36% receiving placebo, $P<0.001$). Remission at week 26 was achieved in 48% of patients in the certolizumab group and in 29% in the placebo group ($P<0.001$).

References

1 Schreiber S, Rutgeerts P, Fedorak RN, et al. A randomized, placebo-controlled trial of certolizumab pegol (CDP870) for treatment of Crohn's disease. *Gastroenterology* 2005; **129**: 807–18.
2 Sandborn WJ, Feagan BG, Stoinov S, et al. Certolizumab pegol for the treatment of Crohn's disease. *N Engl J Med* 2007; **357**: 228–38.
3 Schreiber S, Khaliq-Kareemi M, Lawrance IC, et al. Maintenance therapy with certolizumab pegol for Crohn's disease. *N Engl J Med* 2007; **357**: 239–50.

Index

Abatacept
  clinical trials, 81–88
Adalimumab
  Behçet's disease, 35
  clinical trials
    dermatology, 110
    gastroenterology, 131–134
    rheumatology, 48–56
  clinical use, xiii
  effects on rheumatoid arthritis
    cardiovascular events, 30–31
    combination therapy, 31
    joint damage progression, 30
    little difference between regularly used drugs, 27–30
    switching of blockers, 31
    variable outcomes, 27
  gastroenterology
    administration and dosages, 127–128
    effectiveness, 126
  general safety issues
    allergic reactions, 7–8
    congestive heart failure, 14
    haematology, 18
    injection site reactions, 7
    latent tuberculosis, 5–6
    lupus-like reactions, 12
    neurological diseases, 14–15
    safe use for rheumatoid arthritis, 2
  licensed therapy for psoriasis, 101–102
  treatment of ankylosing spondylitis
    clinical trial measurements, 38–41
    references, 41–44
    scope, 38
  treatment of PsA, 45
Adult Still's disease, 36
Alefacept
  clinical trials, 118–121
  US licensed therapy for psoriasis, 101–102
Allergic reactions, 7–8
Amevive. *see* **Alefacept**
Anakinra
  cancer risk, 10
  clinical trials, 89–92
  use on rheumatoid arthritis, 34
Anaphylactic responses, 7–8
Ankylosing spondylitis
  clinical trial measurements, 38–41
  clinical trials
    etanercept, 64–66
    infliximab, 75–77

  development of psoriasis, 8
  references, 41–44
  scope, 38
Anti-drug antibodies
  abatacept, 87
  general safety issues, 12–13
Arthritis. *see* **Psoriatic arthritis; Rheumatoid arthritis**

B-cell depletion, 93–97
Behçet's disease, 35

Cancer risk
  general safety issues, 9–12
  postmarketing in Crohn's disease, 19
Certolizumab pegol
  anti-drug antibodies, 12–13
  blocking drugs in clinical use, xiii
  clinical trials
    gastroenterology, 148–150
    rheumatology, 79–80
  gastroenterology
    administration and dosages, 128
    effectiveness, 126
Cimzia. *see* **Certolizumab pegol**
Clinical trials
  dermatology
    adalimumab, 110
    alefacept, 118–121
    efalizumab, 113–117
    etanercept, 103–105
    infliximab, 106–109
  gastroenterology
    adalimumab, 131–134
    certolizumab pegol, 148–150
    infliximab, 135–142
    natalizumab, 143–147
  rheumatology
    abatacept, 81–88
    adalimumab, 48–56
    anakinra, 89–92
    B-cell depletion, 93–97
    certolizumab pegol, 79–80
    etanercept, 57–67
    infliximab, 68–78
Congestive heart failure, 13–14
Crohn's disease
  alternative strategies compared, 124–125
  clinical trials
    adalimumab, 131–134
    certolizumab pegol, 148–150

Crohn's disease (*cont.*)
clinical trials (*cont.*)
infliximab, 135–140
natalizumab, 143–147
future directions, 125–126, 126
overview, 122–123
pathogenesis in clinical context, 122–123
safety issues
anti-drug antibodies, 12–13
cancer risk, 11
congestive heart failure, 14
development of psoriasis, 8
hepatitis, 15
neurological diseases, 14–15
postmarketing experience, 18–20
unmet medical needs, 124

Dermatology
clinical trials
adalimumab, 110
alefacept, 118–121
efalizumab, 113–117
etanercept, 103–105
infliximab, 106–109
psoriasis
approaches to management, 99–100
assessing severity, 100
licensed therapies, 101–102
overview, 98–99
references, 103
rheumatoid arthritis distinguished, 101
treatment of PsA, 45

Efalizumab
clinical trials, 113–117
US licensed therapy for psoriasis, 101–102
Enbrel. *see* **Etanercept**
Etanercept
clinical trials
dermatology, 103–105
rheumatology, 57–67
clinical use, xiii
effect on vasculitis, 35
effects on rheumatoid arthritis
cardiovascular events, 30–31
combination therapy, 31
joint damage progression, 30
little difference between regularly used drugs, 27–30
switching of blockers, 31
variable outcomes, 27
general safety issues
allergic reactions, 7–8
cancer risk, 9–12
congestive heart failure, 13–14
effects on lactation, 17
haematology, 18
injection site reactions, 7

lupus-like reactions, 12
neurological diseases, 14–15
use in pregnancy, 16
vaccinations, 17–18
treatment of ankylosing spondylitis
clinical trial measurements, 38–41
references, 41–44
scope, 38
treatment of PsA, 45
US licensed therapy for psoriasis, 101–102

Gastroenterology
alternative strategies compared, 124–125
clinical trials
adalimumab, 131–134
certolizumab pegol, 148–150
infliximab, 135–142
natalizumab, 143–147
references, 129–130
effective therapies, 126
future directions, 125–126
overview, 122–123
pathogenesis in clinical context, 123–124
unmet medical needs, 124
Gout, 36

Haematology
abatacept, 87
general safety issues, 18
Heart failure, 13–14
Hepatitis, 15–16
hepatitis B, 15–16
hepatitis C, 16
increased levels, 15
Humira. *see* **Adalimumab**
Hypersensitivity reactions
abatacept, 87
general safety issues, 7–8

Immunogenicity, 12–13
Infectious diseases
anakinra, 91
B-cell depletion, 96
efalizumab, 114–115
postmarketing in Crohn's disease, 19
respiratory disorders, 17
safety issues
opportunistic infections, 7
tuberculosis, 3–7
Inflammatory bowel disease
administration and dosages, 127–128
alternative strategies compared, 124–125
future directions, 125–126, 126
overview, 122–123
pathogenesis in clinical context, 122–123
unmet medical needs, 124
Infliximab
clinical trials
dermatology, 106–109

gastroenterology, 135–142
rheumatology, 68–78
clinical use, xiii
effect on rheumatological conditions
  Behçet's disease, 35
  sarcoidosis, 36
  vasculitis, 35
effects on rheumatoid arthritis
  cardiovascular events, 30–31
  combination therapy, 31
  joint damage progression, 30
  little difference between regularly used drugs, 27–30
  switching of blockers, 31
  variable outcomes, 27
gastroenterology
  administration and dosages, 127
  effectiveness, 126
general safety issues
  allergic reactions, 8
  anti-drug antibodies, 12–13
  cancer risk, 9–12
  congestive heart failure, 13–14
  hepatitis, 15
  infusion reactions, 8–9
  latent tuberculosis, 6
  lupus-like reactions, 12
  neurological diseases, 14–15
  postmarketing in Crohn's disease, 18–20
treatment of ankylosing spondylitis
  clinical trial measurements, 38–41
  references, 41–44
  scope, 38
treatment of PsA, 45
US licensed therapy for psoriasis, 101–102
Infusion reactions
  abatacept, 87
  B-cell depletion, 96
  general safety issues, 8–9
Injection site reactions
  anakinra, 91
  general safety issues, 7
Isoniazid
  latent tuberculosis, 4–6

Kineret. *see* **Anakinra**

Lactation
  abatacept, 87
  general safety issues, 17
Lenercept, xiv
  allergic reactions, 8
Lupus-like reactions, 12
Lymphoproliferative conditions, 9–12

MabThera
  clinical trials, 93–97

Malignancy conditions
  general safety issues, 9–12
  postmarketing in Crohn's disease, 19

Natalizumab
  administration and dosages, 128
  clinical trials, 143–147
Neurological diseases, 14–15

Orencia. *see* **Abatacept**

Pregnancy
  abatacept, 87
  B-cell depletion, 96
  efalizumab, 116
  general safety issues, 16–17
Psoriasis
  approaches to management, 99–100
  assessing severity, 100
  clinical trials
    adalimumab, 110
    alefacept, 119–120
    efalizumab, 114–117
    etanercept, 103–105
    infliximab, 106–109
  licensed therapies, 101–102
  overview, 98–99
  references, 103
  rheumatoid arthritis distinguished, 101
  safety issues
    allergic reactions, 8
    use with other medications, 18
Psoriatic arthritis
  clinical trials
    etanercept, 62–63
    infliximab, 72–75
  references, 46–47
  safety issues, 46
  scope, 38
  treatment, 44–45

Raptiva. *see* **Efalizumab**
Remicade. *see* **Infliximab**
Respiratory diseases, 17
Rheumatoid arthritis
  B-cell depletion, 33–34
  cardiovascular events, 30–31
  clinical trials
    abatacept, 82–87
    anakinra, 90–91
    B-cell depletion, 94–97
    certolizumab pegol, 79–80
    etanercept, 57
    infliximab, 68–72
  combination therapy, 31
  joint damage progression, 30
  little difference between regularly used drugs, 27–30

Rheumatoid arthritis (*cont.*)
  psoriasis distinguished, 101
  references, 31–33
  safety issues, 2
    anti-drug antibodies, 12–13
    cancer risk, 9–12
    congestive heart failure, 14
    hepatitis, 15
    infectious diseases, 2
    lupus-like reactions, 12
    neurological diseases, 14–15
    psoriasis, 8
    research data, 1
    respiratory disorders, 17
    use with other medications, 18
    vaccinations, 17–18
      switching of blockers, 31
      variable outcomes, 27
Rheumatology
  ankylosing spondylitis
    clinical trial measurements, 38–41
    references, 41–44
    scope, 38
  clinical trials
    abatacept, 81–88
    adalimumab, 48–56
    anakinra, 89–92
    B-cell depletion, 93–97
    certolizumab pegol, 79–80
    etanercept, 57–67
    infliximab, 68–78
  other conditions
    Adult Still's disease, 36
    Behçet's disease, 35
    gout, 36
    overview, 34
    sarcoidosis, 35–36
    Sjögren's disease, 35
    vasculitis, 35
  psoriasis, 41–44
  rheumatoid arthritis
    B-cell depletion, 33–34
    cardiovascular events, 30–31
    combination therapy, 31
    joint damage progression, 30
    little difference between regularly used drugs, 27–30
    references, 31–33
    switching of blockers, 31
    variable outcomes, 27
Rifampicin-isoniazid
  latent tuberculosis, 5
Rituximab
  clinical trials, 93–97
  effect on Sjögren's disease, 35
  effects on rheumatoid arthritis, 33–34

Safety issues
  abatacept, 86–87

  allergic reactions, 7–8
  anakinra, 91
  anaphylactic responses, 7–8
  anti-drug antibodies, 12–13
  B-cell depletion, 96–97
  cancer risk, 9–12
  certolizumab pegol, 80
  congestive heart failure, 13–14
  efalizumab, 116–117
  haematology, 18
  hepatitis, 15–16
  hypersensitivity reactions, 7–8
  infusion reactions, 8–9
  injection site reactions, 7
  lactation, 17
  lupus-like reactions, 12
  neurological diseases, 14–15
  opportunistic infections, 7
  postmarketing in Crohn's disease, 18–20
  pregnancy, 16–17
  PsA, 46
  psoriasis, 8
  references, 20–26
  research data, 1
  respiratory diseases, 17
  risk of infection, 2
  treatment of PsA, 46
  tuberculosis, 3–7
  use with other medications, 18
  vaccinations, 17–18
Sjögren's disease, 35
Still's disease, 36

Tuberculosis
  critical role of TNF, 3
  patient surveillance, 6–7
  response to identification, 4–6
  screening, 3–4
Tumour necrosis factor (TNF)
  active receptors, xi
  blocking drugs
    in clinical use, xiii
    mode of action, xii
    not in clinical use, xiv
  safety issues
    allergic reactions, 7–8
    anaphylactic responses, 7–8
    anti-drug antibodies, 12–13
    cancer risk, 9–12
    congestive heart failure, 13–14
    haematology, 18
    hepatitis, 15–16
    hypersensitivity reactions, 7–8
    infusion reactions, 8–9
    injection site reactions, 7
    lactation, 17
    lupus-like reactions, 12
    neurological diseases, 14–15
    opportunistic infections, 7

postmarketing in Crohn's
  disease, 18–20
pregnancy, 16–17
psoriasis, 8
references, 20–26
research data, 1
respiratory diseases, 17
risk of infection, 2
tuberculosis, 3–7
use with other medications, 18
vaccinations, 17–18
Tysabri. *see* **Natalizumab**

Ulcerative colitis
  alternative strategies compared, 124–125
  clinical trials
    infliximab, 140–141
  future directions, 125–126, 126
  overview, 122–123
  pathogenesis in clinical
    context, 122–123
  unmet medical needs, 124

Vaccinations, 17–18
Vasculitis, 35